Department of Veterans Affairs
Health Services Research & Development Service | Evidence-based Synthesis Program

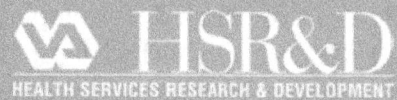

Interventions to Improve Minority Health Care and Reduce Racial and Ethnic Disparities

September 2011

Prepared for:
Department of Veterans Affairs
Veterans Health Administration
Health Services Research & Development Service
Washington, DC 20420

Prepared by:
Evidence-based Synthesis Program (ESP) Center
Portland VA Medical Center
Portland, OR
Devan Kansagara, MD, MCR, Director

Investigators:
Principal Investigator:
  Ana R. Quiñones, PhD

Co-Investigators:
  Maya O'Neil, PhD
  Somnath Saha, MD
  Michele Freeman, MPH
  Stephen R. Henry, DrPH, MPH
  Devan Kansagara, MD, MCR

PREFACE

Health Services Research & Development Service's (HSR&D) Evidence-based Synthesis Program (ESP) was established to provide timely and accurate syntheses of targeted healthcare topics of particular importance to Veterans Affairs (VA) managers and policymakers, as they work to improve the health and healthcare of Veterans. The ESP disseminates these reports throughout the VA.

HSR&D provides funding for four ESP Centers and each Center has an active VA affiliation. The ESP Centers generate evidence syntheses on important clinical practice topics, and these reports help:

- develop clinical policies informed by evidence,
- guide the implementation of effective services to improve patient outcomes and to support VA clinical practice guidelines and performance measures, and
- set the direction for future research to address gaps in clinical knowledge.

In 2009, the ESP Coordinating Center was created to expand the capacity of HSR&D Central Office and the four ESP sites by developing and maintaining program processes. In addition, the Center established a Steering Committee comprised of HSR&D field-based investigators, VA Patient Care Services, Office of Quality and Performance, and Veterans Integrated Service Networks (VISN) Clinical Management Officers. The Steering Committee provides program oversight, guides strategic planning, coordinates dissemination activities, and develops collaborations with VA leadership to identify new ESP topics of importance to Veterans and the VA healthcare system.

Comments on this evidence report are welcome and can be sent to Nicole Floyd, ESP Coordinating Center Program Manager, at nicole.floyd@va.gov.

Recommended citation: Quiñones AR, O'Neil M, Saha S, Freeman M, Henry S, Kansagara D. Interventions to Reduce Racial and Ethnic Disparities. VA-ESP Project #05-225; 2011

This report is based on research conducted by the Evidence-based Synthesis Program (ESP) Center located at the Portland VA Medical Center, Portland OR funded by the Department of Veterans Affairs, Veterans Health Administration, Office of Research and Development, Health Services Research and Development. The findings and conclusions in this document are those of the author(s) who are responsible for its contents; the findings and conclusions do not necessarily represent the views of the Department of Veterans Affairs or the United States government. Therefore, no statement in this article should be construed as an official position of the Department of Veterans Affairs. No investigators have any affiliations or financial involvement (e.g., employment, consultancies, honoraria, stock ownership or options, expert testimony, grants or patents received or pending, or royalties) that conflict with material presented in the report.

TABLE OF CONTENTS

EXECUTIVE SUMMARY
Background 1
Methods 1
Results 2
Summary of Findings 2
Discussion 5

INTRODUCTION
Background 8

METHODS
Topic Development 9
Search Strategy 10
Study Selection, Quality Assessment and Data Abstraction 10
Data Synthesis 11
Peer Review 11

RESULTS
Literature Search 12
Key Question #1. What is the state of research on interventions to reduce race/ethnic disparities or to improve health and health care in minority populations within VA health care settings? 13
Key Question #2. What are the results of interventions (within and outside the VA) to reduce race/ethnic disparities or to improve health and health care in minority populations? 14
Summary of Results across Interventions 27

DISCUSSION
State of Intervention Research 28
Conceptual Framework 29
Future Research and Implications for VA Health Care Settings 31

REFERENCES 34

FIGURES
Figure 1. Literature Flow 12
Figure 2. Conceptual Model – Reach of Interventions 31

APPENDIX A. SEARCH STRATEGY 39

APPENDIX B. INCLUSION/EXCLUSION CRITERIA FOR PRIMARY STUDIES AND REVIEWS 41

APPENDIX C. QUALITY RATING CRITERIA FOR REVIEWS 43

APPENDIX D. EVIDENCE TABLE 44

APPENDIX E. REVIEWER COMMENTS AND RESPONSES 49

EXECUTIVE SUMMARY

BACKGROUND

Racial and ethnic disparities are widespread in the US health care system. A 2007 report from the Veterans Affairs (VA) Health Services Research & Development Service (HSR&D) Evidence-based Synthesis Program (ESP) found disparities were prevalent in a variety of clinical arenas within the Veterans Affairs health care system. The report identified several promising avenues for future interventions designed to reduce racial and ethnic disparities.

The objectives of this review are to describe the state of disparities intervention research within the VA, glean lessons from systematic reviews of intervention research not limited to VA settings, and develop an organizing framework to describe studies in this field of research. This report is also intended to inform future disparities intervention research in the VA, as well as VA policies and programs to reduce disparities.

To accomplish these objectives, we will answer the following key questions:

Key Question #1. What is the state of research on interventions to reduce race/ethnic disparities or to improve health and health care in minority populations within VA health care settings?

Key Question #2. What are the results of interventions (within and outside the VA) to reduce race/ethnic disparities or to improve health and health care in minority populations?

METHODS

We conducted a search for recent primary intervention studies of VA patients in MEDLINE® (PubMed®) (2006 through August 2010) using the search strategy developed for the 2007 VA-ESP report on health disparities. We also conducted a follow-up search for recently published studies by investigators conducting current research during the time of the 2007 report. Due to the large amount of literature on race/ethnic intervention studies conducted outside VA settings, we conducted a search for systematic reviews of intervention studies not limited to VA patients in MEDLINE® (PubMed®), the Cochrane Database of Systematic Reviews (OVID), and PsycINFO® (OVID) (database inception through November 2010). We obtained additional articles from reference lists of pertinent studies. Additional articles were obtained through reviewer feedback following review of the initial draft of this report.

Two reviewers assessed the titles and abstracts identified by the literature search for relevance to the key questions. Two reviewers independently reviewed the articles for inclusion, and discordant results were resolved through discussion and input from a third reviewer. We included studies evaluating the effects of an intervention within (single-race) or between racial/ethnic groups (comparative). We relied on systematic reviews and meta-analyses of intervention studies conducted outside the VA setting (inclusion/exclusion criteria provided in Appendix B). We excluded poor quality reviews as defined by previously developed criteria (Appendix C).

RESULTS

The search for systematic reviews yielded 2,127 citations, and the search for primary VA studies published since the 2007 report yielded 1,290 citations. Following a review of these 3,417 titles and abstracts, we selected 115 articles for further review at the full-text level. We organized the literature addressing key question #1 and key question #2 according to clinical or substantive topic area.

SUMMARY OF FINDINGS

Key Question #1. What is the state of research on interventions to reduce race/ethnic disparities or to improve health and health care in minority populations within VA health care settings?

We found five recently published primary studies of interventions involving minority Veteran populations.[1-5] The populations included in these studies varied. Two were comparative and included black and white Veterans.[1,5] Another two studies were comparative with black, white and Hispanic Veteran populations.[2,4] The final study was single-race and examined Native American Veterans.[3]

The effectiveness of the interventions examined by these studies also varied. Only one of the studies examined is able to conclude that the intervention significantly reduced disparities.[4] One of the studies did not examine the effects of the intervention by race group,[1] one study piloted the acceptability of the intervention in the minority population without evaluating the effects on the outcome,[3] one study found reductions in disparities in intermediate outcomes only[5] and the final study concluded that no significant findings were attributable to the intervention.[2]

Key Question #2. What are the results of interventions (within and outside the VA) to reduce race/ethnic disparities or to improve health and health care in minority populations?

The results from systematic reviews of interventions conducted in settings not limited to the VA are summarized by clinical area below:

Diabetes Interventions

Five good quality systematic reviews of interventions for diabetes mellitus identified studies that were mostly conducted in single-race populations. We also identified one primary intervention study tested on a multiethnic population of Veterans. There was some evidence of benefit for interventions focused on community health workers, care managers, and culturally tailored health education for patients. Provider-focused interventions reported improvements in process measures, although computerized reminders for physicians resulted in negligible or negative results. Studies on the long-term effects of diabetes mellitus interventions on process and outcome measures are lacking. Heterogeneity between studies in subjects, settings, study design, and multiple aspects of the interventions limit the comparisons that can be made across studies. One small single center VA study suggests a telemedicine/care coordination intervention may reduce disparities in black Veterans with diabetes; this finding warrants further research.

Arthritis and Pain Management Interventions

Our search identified one fair quality systematic review examining the effects of behavioral interventions for arthritis in minority and white populations. We also identified one primary study of VA patients evaluating the effects of a decision aid on expected postoperative total knee replacement pain and function levels. The systematic review of behavioral interventions for arthritis found limited evidence from two randomized controlled trials that exercise interventions may be effective in improving differences in pain and disability between white and black patients. In addition, one primary VA study investigating an educational intervention provides evidence of improving knowledge and expectations related to total knee replacement for black patients; however, willingness to consider total knee replacement surgery did not change among either whites or blacks. There remains a need for interventions designed to measure and reduce disparities in the burden of osteoarthritis outcomes.

Preventive and Ambulatory Care Interventions

We identified the greatest number of reviews in preventive and ambulatory care interventions. Fourteen good quality reviews of single-race and comparative studies encompassed several preventive health subtopics, including cancer screening, smoking cessation and physical activity and diet. Little research focused on reducing gaps in screening, treatment and outcomes for minority compared to white adults. Several reviews noted the lack of sufficient number of studies to compare similarly configured interventions or specific components of multifaceted interventions. There is some evidence that community health workers may improve rates of preventive health service utilization. Overall, improvements in preventive and ambulatory care for minorities are inconsistent. The overwhelming majority of reviews focused on improving screening and process of care measures for race/ethnic minorities; there is less research evaluating the effects of interventions on health outcomes.

Cardiovascular Disease Interventions

We identified three systematic reviews that examined cardiovascular health care interventions. Most studies were conducted in single-race populations and could not test the ability of interventions to reduce disparities. Those comparative studies with mixed populations did not test for differential intervention effects based on race/ethnicity. The largest body of literature focused in the areas of hypertension and smoking cessation. On the whole, nurse-based interventions were associated with improvements in proximal health outcomes (e.g., blood pressure, lipid level, body mass index) for minority populations, but the addition of community health workers provided limited gains. Culturally tailored education approaches to lifestyle change interventions appear promising. Several small trials suggest intensive nurse-led multicomponent care management interventions may reduce hospitalization in minority patients with heart failure.

HIV/AIDS Interventions

We identified four good quality comparative and single-race systematic reviews (meta-analyses) that examined the effectiveness of behavioral interventions for HIV and sexually transmitted infection risk reduction among African Americans and Hispanic Americans. No intervention studies were specifically designed to reduce disparities. However, evidence suggests that behavioral interventions can be effective in improving HIV/AIDS service utilization and health care outcomes for African American and Hispanic American populations. A number of studies consistently found that behavioral interventions can reduce risky sex behavior and sexually transmitted infection rates. In particular, gender and culture-specific interventions focused on empowerment were effective in at-risk African American female populations. The reviewed studies did not address organizational barriers and only targeted behavioral intervention efficacy. No studies focused on reducing disparities among Veterans.

Mental Health Interventions

We identified two good quality systematic reviews examining interventions aimed at reducing disparities in mental health care in settings not limited to the VA. Additionally, we found two primary studies conducted within VA settings that addressed mental health care disparities. There is good evidence suggesting that multicomponent chronic disease management interventions including case management strategies and care coordination are helpful in reducing health disparities related to depression. There is insufficient research investigating the effectiveness of culturally tailored psychotherapeutic and preventive interventions in reducing disparities in depression; however, the preliminary evidence in this area indicates that these types of culturally tailored interventions hold promise. No good quality primary studies designed to compare disparities before and after interventions in Veteran populations were identified; however, two primary studies provide some support for the feasibility of using technology-based interventions with ethnic minority Veteran populations. There were no good quality reviews examining disparities reduction interventions for mental health conditions other than depression. There is insufficient evidence for psychopharmacological, psychotherapeutic, and preventive interventions in ethnic minority populations. Preliminary research suggests such interventions can be effective, particularly when they are culturally tailored and include a care coordination or case management component.

Cross-Cutting Interventions

We found five good quality reviews conducted in settings not limited to the VA, as well as one primary VA study of interventions that cut across clinical categories. Of the five reviews, four focus on cultural competence training interventions and one focuses on interventions to improve quality of care delivered in primary care settings. One VA study examined the effects of home-based primary care on improving outcomes for minority Veterans with multiple chronic conditions. No primary studies on cultural competence with VA populations were identified. There is good evidence that cultural competence interventions can improve provider knowledge, attitude, and skills, but there are few good quality studies of effects on patient outcomes. Overall, interventions designed to improve the delivery of care for all patients are effective; however, most studies of interventions to reduce disparities between minority and white patients are characterized by poor quality. One small single-site VA study provides very limited initial evidence that care coordination and multiprofessional home-based primary care programs can improve process of care measures for an African American cohort.

Summary of Results across Interventions

Examination of reviews not limited to VA populations as well as primary VA studies points toward comprehensive interventions garnering more promising results. Although not directly comparable, there were some similar intervention types implemented across clinical areas included in this review. Based on our review, interventions that include personnel (e.g., care managers, community health workers) providing increased connectedness between patients and the health care systems they access offer indications of effective intervention results. Though the strength of evidence is limited by methodological issues, small sample sizes, and the preponderance of studies focused on non-VA populations, the most promising interventions in the various clinical areas reviewed were care coordination, care management, community health workers and culturally tailored education interventions. However, it is interesting to note that at least one review of interventions to reduce HIV/AIDS found that efficacious interventions did not use peer outreach.

DISCUSSION

State of Intervention Research

The intent of this review was to take stock of evidence provided by VA intervention studies designed to reduce race/ethnic disparities among minority Veteran populations. However, few published interventions in VA settings were found in our systematic searches. As a result, we examined intervention studies not exclusive to VA populations because many of the interventions studied – outside of those focused on organizational change in non-integrated health systems – could be potentially informative to VA settings. In general, these reviews from disparate clinical and cross-clinical areas find that a good case can be made for interventions based on case manager-led care coordination efforts, culturally tailored education, and community health workers. However, most interventions were implemented in minority populations only, without a comparison group to determine if the interventions were reduced disparities between minority and white patients.

Our review offers the opportunity to categorize existing disparities research in order to highlight gaps in the literature and provide a framework for describing future interventions. Based on our review, we categorized disparities intervention research studies according to the populations included. Most studies included ***single-race*** or minority-only populations, examining the effect of interventions within a group known to receive lower quality care or have poorer outcomes than the majority white population. Effectiveness documented in such studies provides only indirect evidence that the studied intervention will reduce disparities. Fewer studies were ***comparative*** in nature, including both minority and majority populations and comparing measures in both groups before and after the intervention. Such studies provide direct evidence of an intervention's capacity to reduce disparities. However, studies including minority and majority groups did not always report data stratified by race/ethnicity.

We also categorized interventions, as "generic" or "tailored". The bulk of included studies described ***generic*** interventions, ones that are applied without consideration of group specific needs or preferences. Many of these interventions involved quality improvement efforts or care standardization testing the premise that deficits in care for minority groups might be reduced if care was applied similarly to everyone. In contrast, ***tailored*** interventions describe efforts to address barriers specific to a minority group. Many of these interventions involved specially designed educational materials crafted with specific minority groups in mind (e.g., lessons that address knowledge and health beliefs of minority populations), or community health workers that addressed the special needs of minority patients within their own communities. Community health workers were typically members of those minority communities and therefore understood the context and culture of the population served.

Conceptual Framework

Though the evidence base is overall a limited one, there are common intervention types across clinical areas that suggest promising results. Studies that considered patients in their lived environment were often more promising than those focused strictly on care delivered within health systems. This finding suggests that a framework incorporating home and community context, and the social determinants of health and illness can provide a useful way of thinking about effective interventions to reduce disparities. In this view, race/ethnic disparities in health are seen as driven in part by a broad array of social factors—ranging from education, poverty, and community infrastructure—as well as a complex interplay between these social influences, characteristics of communities and environments where individuals reside, and interactions with providers and health care systems.

Reducing disparities in the care and outcomes of minority Veterans poses special challenges that may require integrating medical care and public health interventions, and linking health systems to communities. Despite operating under an integrated health care system with universal access for Veterans, race/ethnic disparities in care and outcomes remain prevalent in VA settings. Reducing disparities in health care and outcomes will require not only improving equity *within* the health care system but extending beyond the system and into the communities where patients live and work. Health care, in other words, may need to incorporate an understanding of the social determinants of health and extend beyond health care facilities into patient communities. Such an approach is in line with current efforts to make the delivery of health care more patient-centered.

Future Research and Implications for VA Health Care Settings

There are several key steps that may aid in the development, testing, and implementation of disparities interventions that could help fill some of the many identified evidence gaps. First and foremost, continuing the VA policy to consistently collect race and ethnicity information for all Veterans is to be encouraged. The ongoing concerted effort to populate race/ethnicity in the VA data records is a critical step to chronicling progress in reducing disparities for minority Veterans. In addition, there are practical and operational considerations to implementing promising interventions. Identifying optimal characteristics for these interventions is necessary for effective implementation. For example, the use of community health workers was frequently identified as a strategy that holds promise for reaching minority populations. However there is substantial heterogeneity in the composition, training, monitoring, frequency of contact and setting for peer health workers. Identifying optimal characteristics (e.g., training protocols, forms, software) for these interventions is necessary for effective implementation. Documentation and implementation details (including unanticipated challenges and solutions) should be encouraged.

In sum, in order to translate promising directions posed in this review into future research and implementation efforts in the VA, it is necessary to consider the following issues:

- Describe interventions in more detail in order to allow for determination of effective components of interventions. For example, in interventions involving

community health workers and care managers, there was poor specification of the training of those personnel.
- Integrate the use of community health workers into VA settings. This could involve Veteran peer advisors coming from communities where Veterans reside.
- Examine the potential for ongoing large VA demonstration projects in care coordination/care management to improve the health of minority Veterans and reduce disparities.
- Enhance the capacity to tailor patient educational materials to address the specific needs of minority Veterans.
- Consider funding studies explicitly designed to measure pre-post changes in disparities between minority and white Veterans.
- Encourage the inclusion of less well studied minority Veteran groups (i.e., Asian/Pacific Islander and American Indian) in the design and implementation of disparities studies.

Few disparities interventions have been implemented in the VA, and although a few race-specific intervention studies are underway, much more work is needed in this area. The barriers to implementing disparities intervention research in VA care settings are not entirely clear. Future steps emanating from this review will include conducting a survey and interviews of key VA informants to identify barriers to dissemination of interventions, in an effort to provide a better understanding of the obstructions in the VA disparities research pipeline.

EVIDENCE REPORT

INTRODUCTION

BACKGROUND

Racial and ethnic disparities are widespread in the US health care system. A 2007 report from the Portland Evidence-based Synthesis Program (ESP) similarly found disparities were prevalent in a variety of clinical arenas within Department of Veterans Affairs (VA). The report identified several promising avenues for future interventions designed to reduce racial and ethnic disparities. The extent to which such intervention research has been conducted in VA populations is unclear, though our review of published studies suggests disparities intervention research in the VA may be lagging behind research of interventions conducted outside of the VA setting. Furthermore, the approach to disparities interventions may be quite varied, and this may further complicate the development of an organized research agenda within the VA. Identifying challenges to conducting intervention research remain critical steps to informing future VA disparities intervention efforts to reduce disparities and improve health outcomes for minority Veterans.

The objectives of this review are to describe the state of disparities intervention research within the VA, glean lessons from systematic reviews of intervention research not limited to VA settings, and develop an organizing framework to describe studies in this field of research. This work is primarily intended for the Equity Portfolio for the VA Health Services Research & Development (HSR&D), the Veterans Health Administration (VHA) Health System Leadership and the field of race/ethnic disparities researchers, for the purposes of informing future disparities intervention research in the VA as well as VA policies and programs to reduce disparities.

METHODS

TOPIC DEVELOPMENT

The review was requested by the director for the Equity Portfolio of the VA HSR&D and commissioned by the Department of Veterans Affairs Evidence-based Synthesis Program. We relied on individual topic expertise to form the technical expert panel for guiding topic development and reviewing drafts of the report. The objective of this report is to review the evidence that addresses the following key questions:

Key Question #1. What is the state of research on interventions to reduce race/ethnic disparities or to improve health and health care in minority populations within VA health care settings?

Key Question #2. What are the results of interventions (within and outside the VA) to reduce race/ethnic disparities or to improve health and health care in minority populations?

We used the following methods to address these questions:

1) Primary literature review of studies with the following characteristics:

   - Patients: any VA patient population
   - Intervention: any intervention primarily designed to reduce disparities or improve quality of care or outcomes for minority populations
   - Comparator: studies comparing minority to non-minority Veterans as well as studies focusing on outcomes for a targeted minority group of Veterans
   - Outcomes: no intention to limit by outcome
   - Timing: any length of follow-up
   - Setting: VA, inpatient or outpatient

2) Review of systematic reviews and meta-analyses of race/ethnic disparities interventions conducted in VA and non-VA settings.

In addition, discuss the utility of categorizing existing disparities research according to the kinds of populations included in the studies as well as by intervention type to provide an organizing language for the interventions literature.

- Two categories to describe included study populations:
  - **Single-race** or minority-only populations: examined the effect of interventions within a group known to receive lower quality care, or have poorer outcomes, than the majority white population. Effectiveness documented in such studies provides only indirect evidence that the studied intervention will reduce disparities.
  - **Comparative**: included both minority and majority populations and compare measures in both groups before and after the intervention. Such studies provide direct evidence of an intervention's capacity to reduce disparities.

- Two categories for intervention types:
  - **Generic** interventions: applied without consideration of group specific needs or

preferences. Many of these interventions involved quality improvement efforts or care standardization testing the premise that deficits in care for minority groups might be reduced if care was applied similarly for everyone.
- *Tailored* interventions: described efforts to address barriers specific to a minority group. Many of these interventions involved specially designed educational materials crafted with specific minority groups in mind (e.g., lessons that address knowledge and health beliefs of minority populations), or community health workers that addressed the special needs of minority patients within their own communities. Community health workers were typically members of those minority communities and therefore understood the context and culture of the population served.

SEARCH STRATEGY

We conducted a search for recent primary intervention studies of VA patients in MEDLINE® (PubMed®) (2006 through August 2010) using the search strategy developed for the 2007 VA ESP report on health disparities (Appendix A). We also conducted a follow-up search for recently published studies by investigators identified in the 2007 report because they were conducting pending intervention work at the time of that report. Finally, we conducted a search for systematic reviews of intervention studies that are not limited to VA patients in MEDLINE® (PubMed®), the Cochrane Database of Systematic Reviews (OVID), and PsycINFO® (OVID) (database inception through November 2010). We obtained additional articles from reference lists of pertinent studies, and through reviewer feedback following review of the initial draft of this report. All citations were imported into an electronic database (EndNote X2).

STUDY SELECTION, QUALITY ASSESSMENT, AND DATA ABSTRACTION

Two reviewers assessed the titles and abstracts identified by the literature search for relevance to the key questions. Potentially relevant full-text articles were retrieved for further review. Two reviewers independently reviewed the articles for inclusion, and discordant results were resolved through discussion and input from a third reviewer. We included individual studies evaluating the effects of an intervention within or between racial/ethnic groups in VA patients. We relied on systematic reviews and meta-analyses of intervention studies conducted outside the VA setting (inclusion/exclusion criteria provided in Appendix B). We excluded poor quality reviews as defined by previously developed criteria (Appendix C). We also excluded reviews of interventions that were not likely to be applicable to VA settings (i.e., studies focused on reducing financial barriers to access).

From each study, we abstracted information on clinical topic, study methodology, population characteristics including race/ethnicity, types of interventions studied, search dates and number of studies included for systematic reviews.

We dual-reviewed each study for quality and data abstraction. Disagreements were resolved through discussion, and a third investigator was consulted when needed to reach consensus.

DATA SYNTHESIS

We examined intervention studies of both primary studies of VA populations, and systematic reviews conducted in settings not limited to the VA. We organized the literature addressing key question #1 and key question #2 according to clinical or substantive topic area in the Results section including: diabetes mellitus, arthritis and pain management, preventive and ambulatory care, cardiovascular disease, human immunodeficiency virus/auto immune deficiency syndrome (HIV/AIDS), mental health, and cross-cutting interventions.

We developed an abstraction form in order to extract data from included primary studies and systematic reviews. Our syntheses of systematic reviews were qualitative in nature. Because we engaged in reviews of systematic reviews, we relied on the conclusions and syntheses from review authors to a large extent. We gave higher consideration to reviews of good quality, as determined by the quality criteria detailed in Appendix C.

PEER REVIEW

A draft version of this report was sent to the technical expert panel and additional peer reviewers. Their comments and our responses are included in Appendix E.

RESULTS

LITERATURE SEARCH

The search for systematic reviews and meta-analyses yielded 2,127 citations, and the search for primary VA studies published since the 2007 report yielded 1,290 citations. Appendix B details the inclusion/exclusion criteria for study selection. Following a review of these 3,417 titles and abstracts, we selected 115 articles for further review at the full-text level. Of these, we included five primary VA studies and 34 systematic reviews across the various clinical areas (Figure 1). The table in Appendix D provides details about the included studies. We discuss the results by key question in the sections that follow.

Figure 1. Literature Flow

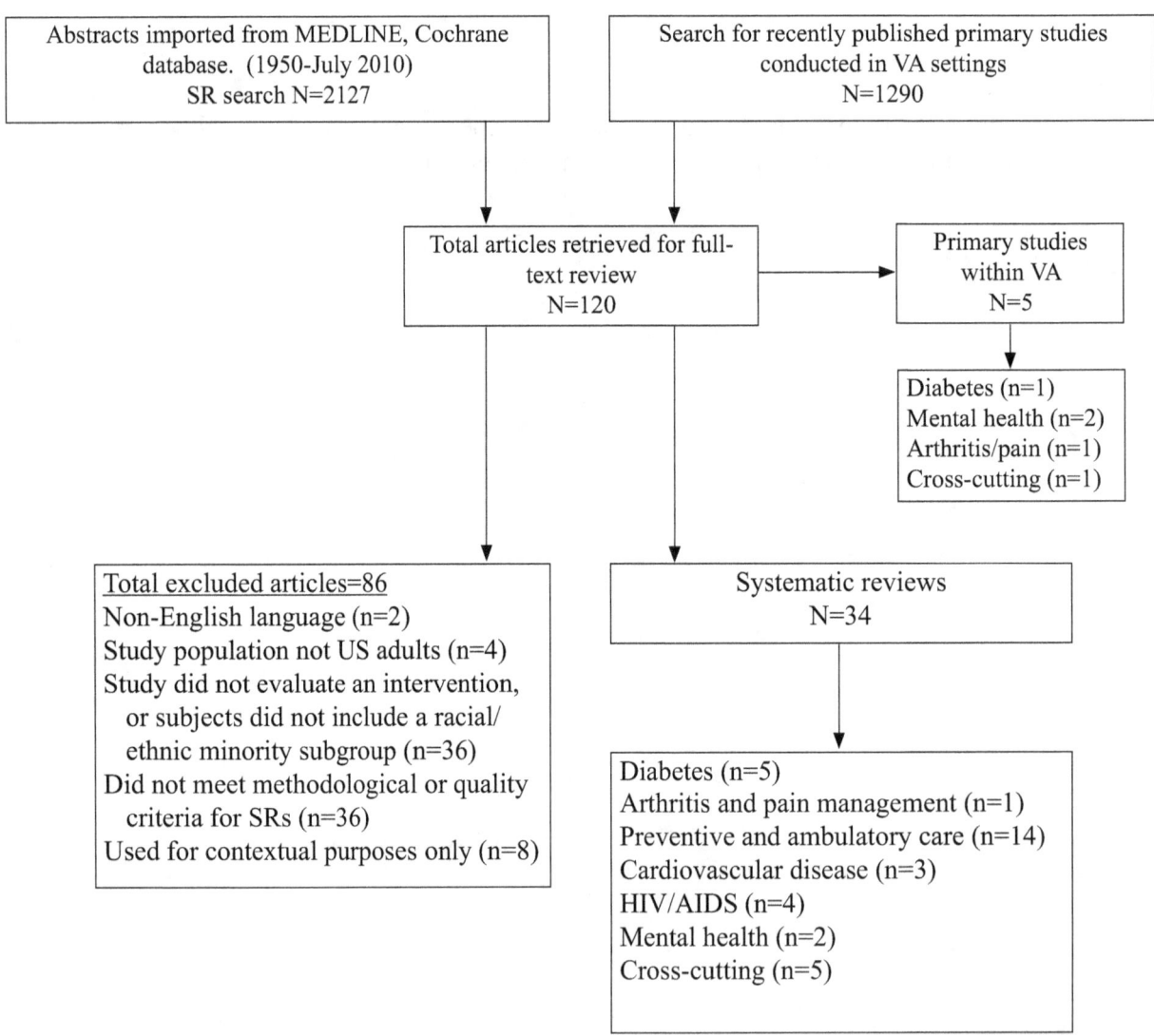

KEY QUESTION #1. What is the state of research on interventions to reduce race/ethnic disparities or to improve health and health care in minority populations within VA health care settings?

We found five recently published primary studies of interventions involving minority Veteran populations.[1-5] The populations included in these studies varied. Two were comparative and included black and white Veterans.[1,5] Another two studies were comparative with black, white and Hispanic Veteran populations.[2,4] The final study was single-race and examined Native American Veterans.[3]

The effectiveness of the interventions examined by these studies also varied. Only one of the studies examined is able to conclude that the intervention significantly reduced disparities.[4] One of the studies did not examine the effects of the intervention by race group,[1] one study piloted the acceptability of the intervention in the minority population without evaluating the effects on the outcome,[3] one study found reductions in disparities in intermediate outcomes only[5] and the final study concluded that no significant findings were attributable to the intervention.[2]

The single-race study compared videoconferencing with in-person administration of a psychiatric assessment among American Indian Vietnam Veterans.[3] Although this study was unable to determine whether the intervention was effective in improving psychiatric outcomes for Native American Veterans, it concluded that teleconferencing was a culturally acceptable method for the delivery of psychiatric care for this sample of minority Veterans. Similarly, one of the comparative studies investigating the effectiveness of a screen-phone assisted care coordination for black, white and Hispanic Veterans with dementia was unable to determine whether the intervention reduced disparities.[2] The study concluded that there were no significant findings. A separate comparative study of black, white and Hispanic Veterans by the same author examined the effects of a phone-based, in-home messaging device combined with care coordination on glycemic control among diabetics.[4] This study was able to conclude that disparities in glycemic control were reduced between white and black Veterans. The fourth study was a comparative study between black and white Veterans that examined the effects of an educational videotape and tailored total knee replacement decision aid on patients' expectations about postoperative pain, physical function, and willingness to consider total knee replacement surgery.[5] This study found decreased disparities between black and white Veterans in intermediate outcomes (knowledge and expectations) rather than in osteoarthritis outcomes. The fifth study was a comparative study between black and white Veterans.[1] The study examined found that the intervention was effective in reducing hospital admissions and total days hospitalized for the study sample, but did not examine the results of the intervention by race.

We discuss the results of each of these primary VA intervention studies in combination with the findings of systematic reviews on similar clinical/substantive topics to key question #2 in the sections that follow.

KEY QUESTION #2. What are the results of interventions (within and outside the VA) to reduce racial/ethnic disparities or to improve health and health care in minority populations?

Diabetes Interventions

Summary

Five good quality systematic reviews of interventions for diabetes mellitus identified studies that were mostly conducted in single-race populations. The outcomes studied included glycemic control measures, patient knowledge and satisfaction, dietary habits, physical activity, self-management activities, emergency room visits and hospital admissions. Process measures included the use of eye exams, microalbumin testing, HbA1c monitoring, foot care, and exercise counseling. We identified a primary intervention study tested on a multiethnic population of Veterans that examined the effects of care coordination and telemedicine intervention on glycemic control. We also reviewed a randomized controlled trial of the effects of cultural competency training on both clinician awareness and glycemic control among black and white outpatients. There was some evidence of benefit for interventions focused on community health workers, care managers, and culturally tailored health education for patients. Provider-focused interventions reported improvements in process measures, although computerized reminders for physicians resulted in negligible or negative results. Studies on the long-term effects of diabetes mellitus interventions on process and outcome measures are lacking. Heterogeneity between studies in subjects, settings, study design, and multiple aspects of the interventions limit the comparisons that can be made across studies. One small single center VA study suggests a telemedicine/care coordination intervention may reduce disparities in black Veterans with diabetes; this finding warrants further research. A study of cultural competency training significantly increased clinician awareness of racial differences in diabetes care, but no effect was observed on reducing disparities between white and black patients on glycemic control targets, LDL cholesterol, or blood pressure 12 months after the intervention.

Details

We identified five good-quality systematic reviews of interventions for diabetes mellitus,[6-11] including a Cochrane review[7] that was subsequently published as a journal article.[6] We found one primary intervention study conducted in VA settings that examined race/ethnic disparities for diabetic Veterans.

The interventions identified by existing reviews included health education interventions;[6,7] the use of community health workers;[10] primary care interventions (including case management, patient counseling, and the use of reminder cards for providers);[9] and self-care interventions aimed to change behavior using culturally tailored techniques.[11] One review included a variety of interventions including patient-targeted interventions, physician provider-targeted interventions, health care organization interventions (including case management, community health workers, and pharmacist-led medication management), and multi-target interventions.[8] Most of the studies identified by the systematic reviews were conducted in single-race populations.

A review of health education interventions determined that culturally tailored health education was more effective than usual care in improving HbA1c and knowledge for up to one year of follow-up, although clinically important long-term outcomes were not examined.[6,7] Another review of health education interventions that sought to improve dietary habits, physical activity, or self-management activities reported that using interpersonal interventions such as peer support and nurses/nutritionists/health educators more often had positive findings than computer-based patient education.[8]

One review examined self-care interventions that aimed to change the behavior of patients, rather than simply educating them. Four of the 12 included studies were designed using cultural tailoring techniques such as the use of focus groups and specific recipes for the ethnic group being studied. Improved glycemic control tended to occur in studies in which baseline glycemic control was markedly poor (A1C>10%). The author of the review concluded that culturally tailored interventions appeared to be successful among African Americans and Latinos, and that self-care interventions may be effective in more difficult-to-treat patients.[11]

One review examined five provider-focused interventions (reminder systems, practice guidelines, continuing medical education, in-person feedback, and problem-based learning) and reported improvements in process measures such as the use of eye exams, microalbumin testing, HbA1c monitoring, foot care, and exercise counseling. By contrast, computerized reminders for physicians resulted in negligible or negative results. None of the physician-targeted studies included provider communication, cultural competence, or shared decision making.[8]

Interventions that used community health workers, care managers, and other non-physician providers showed evidence of benefit, although comparisons across studies were limited by the heterogeneity in the interventions, settings, and types of providers. A review of health care organization interventions found that nurse care managers were effective in improving quality of care as well as patient outcomes, including diabetes control and onset of retinopathy. Telemedicine case management had more modest results than on-site nursing staff. Positive findings were found for other non-physician interventions, including the use of community health workers and medical assistance programs that provided free medications.[8] A review of case management delivered by specialist nurses found improvement in glycemic control and cardiovascular disease risk factors including blood pressure and total cholesterol.[9] A review of community health workers serving in a variety of roles showed some improvements in patient knowledge, behavior and satisfaction, and decreases in emergency room visits and hospital admissions; increases in retinopathy screening and glycemic control monitoring by providers were also noted in a few studies.[10]

A primary study conducted at an urban VA Medical Center (VAMC) examined the effects of a care coordination and telemedicine intervention on glycemic control among older Veteran diabetics.[4] Patients aged 60 and older (mean age 72 years SD=6) were enrolled for at least nine months. Although the study population was small (n=41), it did recruit black (n=14; 34%), white (n=21; 51%) and Hispanic (n=6; 15%) Veterans. The study was designed as a pre-post intervention evaluation. Patients used a telephone-based, in-home messaging device to transmit blood sugar data and answers to clinical questions to the care coordination team, comprised of a nurse practitioner, social worker, administrative assistant, and geriatrician. The data were used to both risk stratify patients and guide ongoing clinical advice from the care coordination team. A comparison of pre- and post-intervention data found that glycemic control improved significantly in black, but not in white or Hispanic Veterans. However, several methodological issues limit the validity of study findings including the single-site observational design and high attrition rate (28 originally eligible Veterans did not complete the study).

Arthritis and Pain Management Interventions

Summary

One fair quality systematic review of behavioral interventions for arthritis in racial and ethnic minority populations found limited evidence from a single randomized controlled trial that exercise interventions may be effective in improving pain and disability. Compared with a health education control program, exercise programs were comparably effective between whites and African Americans in improving pain and disability. In addition, one primary VA study investigating an educational intervention provides evidence of improving knowledge and expectations related to total knee replacement; however, it does not improve willingness to consider total knee replacement surgery.

Details

A fair-quality systematic review[12] that included 25 randomized controlled trials of psychosocial interventions in patients with osteoarthritis or rheumatoid arthritis identified only randomized controlled trial (represented in two publications[13, 14]) that directly compared the effectiveness of an intervention between racial groups. The trial compared an aerobic exercise program and a resistance exercise program with a health education control program; patients were not blinded to the treatment assignment. The study reported that the exercise programs were comparably effective in improving pain and disability between whites and African Americans.

One primary study involved Veterans with moderate to severe knee osteoarthritis. The study assessed whether an educational video and total knee replacement decision aid affected expectations about postoperative pain and physical function following total knee replacement, as well as their willingness to undergo total knee replacement surgery. The study included 31 white and 33 African American Veterans. Although the video and decision aid improved expectations significantly among African American Veterans (bringing them in line with white Veteran expectations), expectations for both groups were still lower than post-total knee replacement outcomes reported by individuals who had undergone total knee replacement surgery. In addition, despite improving knowledge about total knee replacement pain and functional outcomes, the study found little change in participant willingness to consider total knee replacement surgery after the intervention. Although reported baseline and post-intervention willingness runs counter to what is found in previous studies (willingness was higher for African Americans than for white Americans in this study), the educational intervention did not alter subsequent willingness for either group. Despite improving disparities in knowledge and expectations about total knee replacement surgery, this intervention failed to demonstrate a similar improvement in African American Veterans choosing total knee replacement surgery.[5]

Preventive and Ambulatory Care Interventions

Summary

We identified the greatest number of reviews in preventive and ambulatory care interventions. 14 good quality reviews of single-race and comparative studies encompassed several preventive health areas, including cancer screening, smoking cessation, physical activity and diet. Little research explicitly focuses on reducing gaps in screening, treatment and outcomes for minority compared to white adults. Several reviews note the lack of sufficient number of studies to compare similarly-configured interventions or specific components of multifaceted interventions.

There is some evidence that community health workers may improve rates of preventive health service utilization. Overall, improvements in preventive and ambulatory care for minorities are inconsistent. The overwhelming majority of reviews focused on improving screening and process of care measures for race/ethnic minorities; however, there are fewer studies evaluating the effects of interventions on health outcomes.

Details

Eight reviews examined interventions to improve cancer screening rates among various combinations of white, Hispanic, Asian/Pacific Islander, Native American and African American study participants. Two reviews focused on smoking cessation interventions for African Americans and Mexican Americans. Four reviews examined physical activity and diet interventions for African Americans, Hispanics and Japanese Americans. The use of community health workers (also referred to as lay health workers, peer navigators, and *promotoras* in studies among Hispanics), and various examples of culturally tailored health education and counseling were the most commonly evaluated interventions. We found no primary intervention studies conducted in VA settings that examined race/ethnic disparities in preventive and ambulatory care.

Cancer Screening

Eight reviews evaluated interventions designed to improve breast, cervical and colorectal cancer screening and treatment in the United States.[15-22] The best quality breast cancer screening review included 43 studies of primarily African American, Hispanic and white providers and patients.[18] Included studies examined patient-focused (i.e., reminder letters, telephone calls, patient education and counseling), or provider-focused interventions (i.e., clinical reminders, provider education) to improve mammography screening rates. Only two studies examined interventions specifically designed to reduce disparities. These studies found that comprehensive case management interventions that combined health education, counseling, and assistance with health system navigation demonstrated promise in reducing time to initiation of cancer treatment. However, the review also found that interventions aimed at improving screening were more effective for white, educated populations, suggesting that the interventions may exacerbate disparities. Another systematic review also identified health education dissemination for Hispanic women by community health workers to have promising results in improving rates of breast cancer screening.[15]

Three reviews assessed interventions aimed at improving cervical cancer screening.[16, 19, 20] The best and most recent of these reviews examined 18 studies including access enhancement, community education, individual counseling, mass media and community health worker interventions.[20] A meta-analysis of these studies found an overall improvement in cancer screening rates in the intervention groups among African American ($d=0.146$ [95% CI=0.028, 0.265]) and Asian ($d=0.177$ [95% CI=0.098, 0.256]) women, but not among Hispanic ($d=0.116$ [95% CI=-0.008, 0.240]) women. To attempt to explain the neutral findings for Hispanic women, the authors cite potential contamination of treatment and control groups in addition to low education and consequently, low health literacy for this specific ethnic group. Additional analyses found that all intervention types were associated with improvements in Pap screening, with access-enhancing interventions associated with the biggest improvements, while community health workers rendered the smallest effect. The investigators also note that the use of culturally matched materials and culturally matched intervention delivery was associated with improved Pap screening for minority women.

Three reviews examined interventions to increase colorectal cancer screening rates.[19, 21, 22] One review included 15 randomized controlled trials of interventions in multiethnic populations.[22] All interventions were associated with increased screening rates whether they were low intensity outreach programs (i.e., by telephone or mail) or more comprehensive community education programs (i.e., system navigation, risk counseling, cultural self-empowerment). The review found no differences between race/ethnic groups in screening uptake, though five studies did not report outcomes by race/ethnic group in some cases because these data were not collected. Another review offered insights into improving screening among African American patients, such as using personalized materials to educate and remind patients to improve screening adherence.[21] Although this review suggested that the most successful interventions were tailored to address important barriers to screening (i.e., lack of knowledge, perception of risk), the review authors note that only a few studies directly addressed these barriers in the intervention design and evaluated the subsequent effect of interventions on these barriers.

Smoking Cessation

Two good quality reviews offer insights into smoking cessation interventions for minority adults in the US.[23, 24] Each review focused on cessation programs aimed at African American and Hispanic populations, respectively. For African American adults, one meta-analysis of 20 quasi-randomized or randomized controlled trials indicated the odds of quitting were 40 percent higher for intervention programs of stand-alone or combinations of pharmacological, individual/group/telephone counseling, targeted print materials, community outreach and media campaigns, compared to usual care or placebo. Although treatment setting moderated intervention effectiveness (i.e., church and community over clinical settings), treatment intensity did not. Interestingly, culturally specific interventions were only effective insofar as smokers indicated readiness to quit.[23]

One good quality review included in the "Cardiovascular Disease Interventions" section below also examined 13 tobacco cessation intervention trials in minority populations.[25] The findings for that systematic review are largely in agreement with the systematic reviews presented here. In particular, patient-level interventions found that pharmacologic therapy – especially when combined with counseling – was effective in increasing quit rates. Culturally tailored, patient-level interventions produced mixed results. Of note, one study tested physician training and patient enrollment in a culturally tailored cessation program and found a 21 percent quit rate at seven months. Another study found culturally tailored health education was more effective than motivational interviewing.

A systematic review and meta-analysis of 17 studies involving Mexican Americans also indicated good evidence for pharmacological, and moderate evidence for community health workers (*promotoras*) and counseling (both group and telephone) interventions for smoking cessation. However, concerns with methodological design, length of follow-up and generalizability to other Hispanic subgroups limit conclusions based on these findings.

Physical Activity and Diet

Four reviews involved interventions to improve physical activity and nutritional education among minorities.[26-29] We identified one systematic review as the most comprehensive and best quality.[26] This review included 29 studies in African American populations, 15 of which were randomized controlled trials. Intervention modalities included telephone counseling, community health worker counseling, structured exercise programs, group exercise sessions and unstructured exercise programs. Most of the trials found a neutral effect of interventions. Those interventions that were associated with benefit demonstrated only short-term improvements in physical activity behavior change.

A second review of 19 culturally tailored weight loss intervention trials in African American, Hispanic, and Japanese American adults found that though most found a benefit from the intervention, the benefits were short-lived.[27] The authors also indicate that even the short-term weight loss benefits did not extend to African American women.

In a third review, tailored nutrition programs showed marginal benefit, although there were few studies that examined race/ethnic group differences explicitly and little exposition of tailored education program details.[28] This meta-analysis included multiple ethnic groups, including white, African American and Hispanic adults in 16 quasi- or randomized controlled trials. Tailored nutrition education interventions were implemented in the form of face-to-face interactions, email or print materials and appear effective in improving dietary intake over the long-term (six months or more) for priority minority groups. However, review authors do not comment on minority versus white intervention effectiveness.

One review focused on Hispanic Americans and found the use of community health workers (*promotoras*) for peer nutrition education improved diabetes disease management, though the authors emphasize the need for longer-term trials to further evaluate the effectiveness of such interventions.[29]

Cardiovascular Disease Interventions

Summary

We identified three systematic reviews that examined cardiovascular health care interventions. Most studies were conducted in single-race populations and could not test the ability of interventions to reduce disparities. Those comparative studies with mixed populations did not test for differential intervention effects based on race/ethnicity. The largest body of literature focused in the areas of hypertension and smoking cessation. On the whole, nurse-based interventions were associated with improvements in proximal health outcomes (e.g., blood pressure, lipid level, body mass index) for minority populations, but the addition of community health workers provided limited gains. Culturally tailored education approaches to lifestyle change interventions appear promising. Several small trials suggest intensive nurse led multicomponent care management interventions may reduce hospitalization in minority patients with heart failure.

Details

We found three systematic reviews examining interventions related to cardiovascular health.[25,30,31] The Davis et al. review was methodologically the most rigorous of these, and included studies from 1995 to 2006 of a broad variety of health care delivery interventions focusing on cardiovascular risk factor management (hypertension, hyperlipidemia, smoking, obesity), and management of cardiovascular conditions including myocardial infarction and heart failure. Studies were included if they included >50 percent minority populations, or were subgroups of larger trials for which race/

ethnicity subgroup data were reported. Studies were excluded if the intervention had no connection to a health care setting. Most studies included minority-only populations and therefore could not test the impact of the interventions on disparities. The authors did find, however, a number of interventions tested in minority populations summarized below:

- Twenty-seven studies of interventions focused on hypertension, most of which were intended to change the structure of care delivery. Only nine studies evaluated patient-level interventions. Nursing interventions – either using home nurses alone or in combination with community health workers – were assessed in eight studies, most of which found these interventions to be successful in lowering blood pressure. Some of these also successfully lowered lipid levels. Pharmacist and community health worker interventions were not well studied. One clinic reorganization intervention was effective for both African Americans and whites, while two others were either ineffective or demonstrated only short-term gains. Of note, one of these was a VA study which found that chart-based reminders failed to improve physician adherence to hypertension guidelines. Patient-level interventions such as salt restriction were effective in some studies, and the Dietary Approaches to Stop Hypertension diet was significantly more effective in African Americans than in other racial/ethnic groups.
- Four patient-level hyperlipidemia intervention studies produced largely negative results, though studies using culturally tailored recipes in African Americans did find very modest improvements in lipid levels.
- The review included 13 trials examining tobacco cessation interventions in minority populations, and these results are described under the "prevention" section above.
- Only three trials assessed interventions promoting physical activity; high drop-out rates limited the conclusions that could be drawn from these studies.
- Four trials found nurse-led care management interventions featuring patient education and close follow-up appeared to reduce heart failure hospitalizations in minority subpopulations.

One poor quality review, which covers an identical search period as Davis et al., did not present study results, but included a qualitative critique of the literature.[30] The authors' interpretation of the literature indicated that the location of health care delivery matters, with community based approaches being particularly promising. They also noted that studies did not clearly show intensive interventions to be more effective than less intensive ones, and the intensity of intervention may have contributed to the high attrition rates seen in some studies. They noted that group based interventions were associated with high rates of recruitment and retention.

Finally, a third review focused on Native Hawaiian and other Pacific Islander populations and found only three intervention studies which were all limited by significant methodological weaknesses.[31]

HIV/AIDS Interventions

Summary

No intervention studies were specifically designed to reduce disparities. However, evidence suggests that behavioral interventions can be effective in improving HIV/AIDS service utilization and health care outcomes for African American and Hispanic populations. A number of studies consistently found that behavioral interventions can reduce risky sex behavior and sexually transmitted infection rates. In particular, gender and culture specific interventions focused on empowerment were effective in at-risk African American female populations. The reviewed studies did not address organizational barriers and only targeted behavioral intervention efficacy. Based on this scant evidence, there is insufficient data to suggest that these interventions would be effective in reducing disparities in HIV/AIDS. Moreover, none of the reviews focus on reducing disparities among Veterans.

Details

We identified four good quality meta-analytic reviews that examined behavioral interventions to reduce HIV risk behaviors and incidence of sexually transmitted infections among African Americans and Hispanic Americans. None evaluated the effectiveness of behavioral HIV/sexually transmitted infection risk reduction interventions in reducing racial and ethnic disparities in HIV service utilization or health outcomes between racial/ethnic groups.

One systematic review evaluated the efficacy of HIV behavioral interventions for African American women.[32] The majority of participants were low income women who were unemployed or received public assistance. Most studies contained multiple intervention components aimed at reducing the risk of heterosexual transmission of HIV. All interventions provided information to increase HIV/sexually transmitted infection knowledge. Skills training components usually took specific forms, including correct use of male condoms, or negotiating safer sex practices through demonstration or role-playing. Several common constructs of behavioral change theories were addressed, including motivation; positive attitude toward condoms; normative influence; self-efficacy for protective behavior; personal responsibility to protect oneself, family, significant others, or community; and personal risk or vulnerability. Most interventions were delivered in small groups, had more than one session, and lasted longer than 240 minutes.

In 33 studies including 11,239 patients, interventions overall reduced unprotected sex rates by 37 percent (OR=0.63; 95% CI=0.54 - 0.75), and in 17 studies interventions reduced sexually transmitted infection diagnosis rates by 19 percent (OR=0.81; 95% CI=0.67, 0.98; n=8760). Efficacious interventions were those delivered by women, and focused on self-efficacy, assertiveness, and negotiation skills intended to empower women to seek equality in their relationships. Additionally, the success of HIV behavioral risk interventions may be more dependent on the quality than number of intervention sessions. Culturally tailored interventions with fewer sessions and skills training were as efficacious as multiple session interventions in reducing HIV risk behaviors.

Another systematic review by the same author evaluated the efficacy of behavioral interventions in reducing unprotected sex and sexually transmitted infection incidence among African American and Hispanic American sexually transmitted infection clinic patients, and found similar positive results.[33] The number of intervention sessions ranged from one to eight, were commonly delivered in small groups, took 10 minutes to 16 hours to deliver, and spanned from less than one day to six months. Beneficial intervention effects were seen in trials regardless of participants' characteristics (i.e., sexually transmitted infection date at baseline, specifically targeting African Americans or Hispanic Americans, 90 percent of participants being African American or Hispanic American), methodological quality of trials (i.e., participation rate, retention rate, reporting generation of randomization sequence or allocation concealment), or intervention features (e.g., intervention contents or setting, unit of delivery, total time to deliver intervention). In addition, the review found that interventions using facilitators that were ethnically matched to patients were more efficacious.

Despite being of lower quality, we included the third review to provide limited discussion of the effectiveness of behavioral interventions in reducing HIV transmission among African Americans.[34] The analyses indicated that, overall, sexual risk reduction intervention participants improved condom use but neither increased nor decreased the number of sexual partners compared with controls. Interventions less than 13 weeks long achieved greatest results when the intervention content included intrapersonal skills training (i.e., self-management). Interventions lasting from 13 to 43 weeks were more effective when the interventions included: (a) more HIV+ participants or men who have sex with men and fewer intravenous drug users, (b) higher retention rates, (c) tailored content to participants, (d) more sessions of longer duration, (e) interpersonal skills training (i.e., partner negotiation), and (f) no counseling and testing. Interventions of longer duration (i.e., 43 to 152 weeks) were more effective when they: (a) included a sampling of more HIV+ participants, younger people, and females; (b) had higher retention rates; (c) tailored content to participants; (d) offered more sessions; (e) included interpersonal skills training; and (f) did not include counseling and testing.

The fourth review focused on HIV/AIDS or sexually transmitted infection prevention interventions seeking to reduce the HIV risk behaviors of Hispanic Americans residing in the US or Puerto Rico.[35] In summary, participants in the intervention groups experienced a 25 percent reduced odds of engaging in sex risk behaviors (OR = .75, 95% CI = .66–.85); a 56 percent increased odds of condom use (Reverse =1.56; OR = .64, 95% CI = .54–.75); a 25 percent reduced odds of unprotected sexual intercourse (OR = .75, 95% CI = .63–.89); a 25 percent reduced odds of number of sex partners (OR = .75, 95% CI = .66–.86); a 31 percent reduced odds of new sexually transmitted infections (OR = .69, 95% CI = .54–.88); a 17 percent reduced odds of engaging in injection drug use; and a 27 percent reduced odds of sharing injection paraphernalia (OR = .73, 95% CI = .63–.85). Efficacious interventions: (a) did not use peer outreach, $p < .01$; (b) were delivered by non-peers such as health care providers, counselors or other professional facilitators, $p < .05$; (c) comprised of four or more sessions, $p < .05$; (d) included problem solving skills, $p < .01$; (e) discussed barriers to condom use, $p < .01$ and sexual abstinence, $p < .05$; (f) used peer norms to encourage behavior change, $p < .05$.; and (g) targeted either females only or males only and were successful in reducing sex risk behavior, $p < .01$. Interventions that utilized ethnographic formative interviews, $p < .05$, or addressed the Hispanic traditional gender norm of machismo, $p < .05$, were more efficacious than those that did not.

Mental Health Interventions
Summary
There is good evidence suggesting that multicomponent chronic disease management interventions including case management strategies and care coordination are helpful in reducing health disparities related to depression. There is insufficient research investigating the effectiveness of culturally tailored psychotherapeutic and preventive interventions in reducing

depression health disparities; however, the preliminary evidence in this area indicates that these types of culturally tailored interventions hold promise. No good quality primary studies designed to reduce health disparities in Veteran populations were identified; however, two primary studies provide initial support for the feasibility of using technology-based interventions with ethnic minority Veteran populations. There were no good quality reviews examining disparities reduction interventions for mental health conditions other than depression. Though there is insufficient evidence for psychopharmacological, psychotherapeutic, and preventive interventions in ethnic minority populations, preliminary research on a variety of interventions suggests that such interventions can be effective for this population, particularly when they are culturally tailored and include a care coordination or case management component.

Details

We identified two good quality systematic reviews examining interventions aimed at reducing health disparities in mental health care in settings not limited to the VA. Additionally, we found two primary studies conducted within VA settings that addressed mental health care disparities interventions.

One systematic review examined 20 interventions related to depressive disorders.[36] Of the 20 reviewed interventions, 14 were randomized controlled trials and six were observational studies. This group of studies was comprised of 12 studies which the authors classified as "chronic disease management" research including case management and collaborative care approaches; the remaining eight were classified as "culturally tailored interventions" and included treatment programs, preventive interventions, and psychoeducation.

Multicomponent chronic disease management interventions were successful in reducing or eliminating disparities; in most cases, ethnic minorities obtained a greater benefit than non-Hispanic white participants, though outcomes for minority populations often remained below those of majority group. The authors identified the following components of successful chronic disease management interventions: practice redesign, patient education, expert consultation or decision support, feedback information, active case management by a trained provider or layperson, and adequate tailoring to patient and provider unique factors. Systems-level interventions included enhanced access to care (including patient cost reduction as well as integrated mental/physical health care), screening, and process improvements (including meetings, patient reminders, progress reviews, and expert team leaders). It was generally impossible to identify the individual parts of these multicomponent interventions that were more or less efficacious. However, physician reminders and screening tools alone were not effective in reducing disparities. Among patient-level intervention studies, case management was the most commonly used strategy. Case management was provided by a range of providers and laypersons, and focused on improved access and adherence to care, mental health care stigma, and psychotherapy focused on management of challenges; this was often accompanied by reading, electronic, and culturally tailored educational materials.

Culturally tailored psychotherapy and preventive interventions were described as showing promise, though few randomized controlled trials were identified. Promising components of cultural tailoring included culturally specific explanatory models of illness (e.g., family structure, autonomy, and time), educational and intervention materials, problem-solving approaches, recruitment of participants, and participant or provider ethnicity (e.g., ethnicity specific groups or providers).

A second systematic review examined 10 studies (7 of which were randomized controlled trials) investigating the effectiveness of psychopharmacological management, psychotherapy, and combination psychotherapy and religion or psychotherapy and case management interventions.[37] There was inconsistent evidence for relative effectiveness of one type of intervention versus another within or across ethnic groups. The authors highlight specific examples of differential response to treatment across ethnic groups, and though group differences were inconsistent across studies, there was consistent evidence supporting the effectiveness of psychotherapeutic and psychopharmacological interventions in ethnic minority populations, particularly when included as part of a case management or care coordination intervention.

In spite of evidence supporting the effectiveness of these interventions in ethnic minority groups, there was inconsistent and insufficient evidence documenting reductions in health disparities related to depression. Many interventions were conducted with only ethnic minority populations, making comparisons to majority group populations impossible. Though some interventions examined multiple ethnic groups, the findings across studies were inconsistent in terms of relative effectiveness of particular intervention types for specific ethnic groups.

We identified two primary intervention studies focused on mental health disparities reduction in Veteran populations. One study investigated a screen-phone assisted care coordination intervention for caregivers of Veterans with dementia.[2] Caregivers were provided with a screen-phone that included visual resources related to caregiving for individuals with dementia, as well as at least monthly phone calls from a nurse care coordinator. Outcomes including burden, depression, coping, quality of life, knowledge, and satisfaction with the intervention were assessed pre- and post-enrollment. There was no control group. The only significant difference on pre-test measures for African American versus white participants was related to burden, with African American participants endorsing significantly more burden than white participants. There were no significant changes on any outcomes comparing pre- and post-test scores. Results related to intervention satisfaction presented in aggregate format across racial/ethnic groups indicated patient satisfaction with the intervention, with 92 percent of participants recommending the intervention. Finally, cost analyses indicated a significant cost savings to the VA of approximately 50 percent compared to pre-intervention service utilization costs.

The other primary study investigated the acceptability of videoconferencing versus in person administration of a psychiatric assessment with an American Indian Veteran population.[3] Though this study did not investigate an intervention, we chose to include it because it investigated a novel method of service delivery designed to reduce mental health disparities in an ethnic minority, Veteran population. This study used a no-control, test-retest design. American Indian participants were administered a culturally tailored, structured clinical interview over videoconferencing and in person. There were no statistically significant differences between the two methods of administration on process and satisfaction measures, though 45 percent of participants indicated a preference for the in-person interview, while only 20 percent indicated a preference for the videoconferencing.

Cross-Cutting Interventions

Summary

There is good evidence that cultural competence interventions can improve provider knowledge, attitude, and skills, but there are few good quality studies of effects on patient outcomes. Overall, interventions designed to improve the standardized delivery of care for all patients are effective; however, most interventions to reduce disparities between minority and white patients are characterized by poor quality. One small single-site VA study provided very limited initial evidence that care coordination and multiprofessional home-based primary care programs can improve process of care measures for an African American cohort.

Details

We found five good quality reviews conducted in settings not limited to the VA,[38-42] as well as one primary VA study[1] concerning interventions that cut across clinical categories. Of the five reviews, four focused on cultural competency interventions and one focused on interventions to improve quality of care delivered in primary care settings. One VA study examined the effects of home-based primary care on improving outcomes for Veterans with multiple chronic conditions.

Cultural Competence Interventions

We identified four good quality systematic reviews investigating the effectiveness of cultural competence interventions. One review examined whether cultural competence interventions improved provider knowledge, attitudes, and skills; as well as patient adherence, satisfaction, and health status outcomes.[41] This review identified 34 studies: 2 randomized controlled trials; 12 non-randomized controlled trials; and 20 non-randomized, non-controlled, pre-post studies. All but three of the included studies focused on provider outcomes and found good evidence that both general and culture-specific cultural competence training improved provider knowledge. There was consistent, fair-quality evidence that cultural competence training improved provider attitudes including cultural self-efficacy, attitudes toward community health issues, and interest in learning about patient and family backgrounds. There was consistent, fair-quality evidence that cultural competence training improved provider skills, including outcomes such as communication skills, community involvement, social interactions, and facility of treatment implementation.

A more recent review focused specifically on patient outcomes and identified seven studies with patient outcomes, including satisfaction, self-efficacy, health status, and patient assessment of provider competence.[38] The studies ranged from poor to fair quality and included two quasi-randomized, two cluster randomized, and three pre-post study designs; four of the studies included in this review were not included in the Beach, 2005 review[41] and investigated outcomes including patient satisfaction, resourcefulness, service access, health status, trust, ratings of physician cultural competence, and treatment adherence. The authors indicate that in spite of low quality and inconsistent results among existing studies, the general trend among studies suggests the potential for cultural competence training to have a positive impact on patient outcomes.

Another review examined comparative interventions designed to facilitate culturally competent health care including as outcomes patient satisfaction, service utilization, and health status.[42] No studies on recruitment and retention of ethnically diverse providers were identified. Two studies provided insufficient evidence for the effectiveness of interpreter/bilingual services in improving patient treatment receipt and adherence. One study provided insufficient evidence for the effectiveness of cultural competence training in improving patient treatment adherence. Four studies provided insufficient evidence for the effectiveness of culturally tailored educational materials in improving treatment receipt and adherence, as well as in terms of patient satisfaction. No studies on culturally specific health care settings were identified.

One review investigated cultural competence interventions in mental health care with a specific focus on evaluation of cultural competence models, and found only nine poor quality observational studies.[39] Overall, evidence for the effectiveness of cultural competence models in mental health care was insufficient and low quality.

Two well-designed randomized controlled trials identified by our technical expert panel may provide additional insights about culturally sensitive approaches to interventions. One study found that culturally tailored peer mentoring on advance directives elicited a significant impact on advance directives completion among black end-stage renal dialysis patients. By contrast, peer mentoring had no effect on advance directives completion among white end-stage renal dialysis patients in the trial.[43] Another randomized controlled trial found that providing clinicians with data reports on disparities along with cultural competency training significantly increased their awareness of racial differences in diabetes care, but there was no effect on reducing disparities between white and black patients on glycemic control targets, LDL cholesterol, or blood pressure 12 months after the intervention.[44] The findings of this study suggest that cultural competence training for clinicians, while effective in raising clinician awareness, may not be sufficient to have a measurable impact on disparities in health outcomes.

Quality Improvement

One good quality systematic review examined health system organization elements, as well as provider education efforts to improve rates of preventive services and quality of care for racial/ethnic minorities.[40] Consisting of 27 studies (20 were randomized controlled trials and seven were case-control studies) predominantly in primary care settings, the authors found mixed evidence regarding various intervention components. Tracking and reminder systems were very effective in increasing rates of preventive service use, particularly for cancer screening and advance directives. However, these effects weren't demonstrated for all clinical areas, limiting their potential for addressing overall disparities.

The review authors identify several additional promising interventions. These include interventions that bypass the physician to offer standardized services directly to patients, use of remote simultaneous translation for patients with limited English proficiency, and using structured questionnaires of patients to assess health behavior risk. Fair evidence was found for bypassing physicians in order to provide preventive services to patients. However, there are no indications that language proficiency may be a relevant issue for Veteran populations; therefore, remote simultaneous translation services may not be applicable to VA settings. The authors also note the dearth of studies to explicitly evaluate the ability of interventions to reduce disparities between minority and white patients.

Home-Based Primary Care

In one primary study, 130 African American (71%) and 53 white (29%) Veterans from an urban VA setting were enrolled in home-based primary care for at least six months.[1] The home-based primary care program involved a multiprofessional team including a medical director, nurse practitioners, registered nurses, social workers, pharmacists, a registered dietician, a dental hygienist and a program director. The single-site study was designed as a retrospective chart review of enrollees, with pre-post intervention evaluation of a number of physical and mental health measures.

Patients were older (mean age 73.6), mostly male (95.6%) and had an average of six comorbidities per patient. The intervention was associated with a significant decrease in hospital admissions (43.7% reduction, p=0.001) and total number of days hospitalized (49.9% reduction, p=0.001), but not in emergency room use. Unfortunately, the study did not analyze outcomes according to race/ethnic group and though the results for this majority African American patient population were encouraging, the intervention's impact on health disparities reduction is uncertain.[1]

SUMMARY OF RESULTS ACROSS INTERVENTIONS

Although not directly comparable, there were some similar intervention types implemented across clinical areas included in this review. Based on our review, interventions that include personnel (e.g., care managers, community health workers) providing increased connectedness between patients and the health care systems they access offer indications of effective intervention results. Though the strength of evidence is limited by methodological issues, small sample sizes, and the preponderance of studies focused on non-VA populations, the most promising interventions in the various clinical areas reviewed were care coordination, care management, community health workers and culturally tailored education interventions. However, it is interesting to note that at least one review of interventions to reduce HIV/AIDS found that efficacious interventions did not use peer outreach.

On balance, efforts to improve quality of health care were largely successful. Various reviews and primary studies detail a narrowing of many gaps in illness care, particularly in the process measures that are the direct responsibility of health care systems and providers. Still, many of the reviewed studies include single-race populations or do not report improvements in minority groups relative to white groups. Therefore, it is difficult to surmise that intervention-specific improvements offer consistent evidence of improved race/ethnic equity in care.

Several reviews discuss effectiveness of organizational interventions that appear specific to less-integrated health systems than the VA. Although these interventions generally garner large effects, there may be only small benefits to implementing these changes into VA health care practice, where the organizational changes are already in place. For example, clinical reminders for both providers and patients had substantial effects for improving uptake of a broad array of preventive services; however, there may be only marginal benefit to VA testing and adoption of these strategies since the VA already extensively uses reminders. Additionally, a variety of interventions tested in settings not limited to the VA rely largely on exploiting the gains from providing access to care for the uninsured. Although financial access to care is not as relevant to VA patient populations, further expansion of access to Veterans residing in areas lacking necessary providers via telehealth practice adoption and availability of community based outreach may have the capacity to reduce race/ethnic disparities in the VA health care system.

DISCUSSION

STATE OF INTERVENTION RESEARCH

The original intent of this review was to take stock of evidence provided by VA intervention studies designed to reduce race/ethnic disparities among minority Veteran populations. However, very few published interventions in VA settings were found in our systematic searches. As a result, we examined intervention studies not limited to VA populations because many of the interventions studied – outside of those focused on organizational change in non-integrated health systems – could be potentially informative to VA settings. Because of the number of studies and the adequacy of existing systematic reviews, we conducted a review of systematic reviews rather than of original studies. The review of reviews also allowed us to discern lessons through a qualitative "meta-synthesis" of the syntheses offered in the existing reviews. In general, these reviews from disparate clinical and cross-clinical areas find that a good case can be made for interventions based on case manager-led care coordination efforts, culturally tailored patient education, and community health workers. However, most studies included only single-race, minority populations. Very few interventions tested for reductions in disparities between minority and white adults. Thus, much of the evidence in the reviews provided only indirect evidence of the potential for interventions to reduce disparities. Fewer interventions still have been tested with Veteran populations.

Our review provided the opportunity to categorize existing disparities intervention research into a framework that can be used to guide future research. This framework builds on a taxonomic system widely used to sort disparities research into three generational categories.[45, 46] First generation research is the term coined for work that identifies race/ethnic disparities in health or health care. In logical sequence, second generation research then attempts to explain and elucidate reasons for these disparities, and third generation work describes efforts to deploy interventions to reduce and eliminate observed disparities. Increased attention to third generation research is seen as a necessary next step in order to continue to make advances in reducing disparities in health and health care. However, little effort has been paid to further categorizing third generation research.

We categorize existing disparities research in order to highlight gaps in the literature and provide a framework for describing future interventions. Based on our review, we categorized disparities intervention research studies according to the populations included. Most studies included *single-race* or minority-only populations, examining the effect of interventions within a group known to receive lower quality care or have poorer outcomes than the majority white population. Effectiveness documented in such studies provides only indirect evidence that the studied intervention will reduce disparities. Fewer studies were *comparative* in nature, including both minority and majority populations, and comparing measures in both groups before and after the intervention. Such studies provide direct evidence of an intervention's capacity to reduce disparities. However, studies including minority and majority groups did not always report data stratified by race/ethnicity.

We also categorized interventions, as "generic" or "tailored". The bulk of included studies described *generic* interventions, ones that are applied without consideration of group specific needs or preferences. Many of these interventions involved quality improvement efforts, or care standardization, testing the premise that deficits in care for minority groups might be reduced if care was applied similarly for everyone. In contrast, *tailored* interventions describe efforts to address barriers specific to a minority group. Many of these interventions involved specially designed educational materials crafted with specific minority groups in mind (e.g., lessons that address knowledge and health beliefs of minority populations), or community health workers that addressed the special needs of minority patients within their own communities. Community health workers were typically members of those minority communities and therefore understood the context and culture of the population served.

Only studies that examine intervention effectiveness with a minority population (or several) alongside whites can detail the extent of a disparity and the potential for the intervention to reduce it. Ideally, these studies would report differences between minorities and whites before and after intervention implementation. Instead, the majority of third generation literature is populated with studies that either: (1) do not allow determination of the presence of a disparity because of the lack of a white comparison group, or (2) do not provide pre-post intervention measures for both minority and white population groups. In order to determine whether interventions are effective in *reducing* disparities in outcomes or care, it is necessary to examine both minority and white populations using a difference-in-difference approach to evaluating intervention effectiveness. However, the methodological challenges (e.g., sample size, ability to receive funding, cost) inherent in designing, testing and implementing interventions to reduce disparities raise questions of feasibility. It is possible that partnering with large projects to investigate multiple research objectives could provide sufficiently large populations of minority Veterans to detect effects in clinically meaningful outcomes.

CONCEPTUAL FRAMEWORK

Though the evidence base is overall a limited one, there are common intervention types across clinical areas that suggest promising results. A key theme was that studies that considered patients in their lived environment were often more promising than those confined to health care systems or interactions. This finding, along with emerging thought about the key drivers of disparities in health and health care, indicates that an intervention framework that considers not only medical care but also incorporates social determinants of health and illness could be helpful in guiding future research. In this view, race/ethnic disparities in health are seen as driven in part by a broad array of social factors – including education, poverty, and community infrastructure – as well as a complex interplay between these social and cultural influences, characteristics of communities and environments where individuals reside, and interactions with providers and health care systems.

Disparities in health and disparities in health care have traditionally been viewed as distinct problems with different solutions. Addressing health disparities has accordingly been viewed largely as a social and public health agenda, beyond the purview of health care delivery systems. Disparities in health care, in contrast, reflect the observation that the quantity and quality of health services received by racial and ethnic minority groups are consistently lower than for the majority white population. Initiatives to address health care disparities typically focus on ensuring equity in health care delivery, which is viewed as a responsibility of health systems.

The role of health systems in addressing social determinants has been limited, with difficulties in dealing with factors that traditionally lie outside of physician purview often cited as a main obstacle.

However, reducing disparities in the care and outcomes of minority Veterans poses special challenges that will require taking down the partition between medical care and public health, and between health systems and communities. Minority Americans bear a disproportionate burden of morbidity and mortality attributable to chronic illnesses, such as diabetes, hypertension and heart disease.[47-49] Despite the fact that the VA provides an integrated health care system with universal access for Veterans, race/ethnic disparities in care and outcomes have been extensively documented in VA settings.[50] Reducing disparities in health care and outcomes will require not only improving equity *within* the health care system, but extending beyond the system and into the communities where patients live and work. VA health care, in other words, may need to incorporate an understanding of the social determinants of health and extend beyond the health care center into patient communities.[51-53]

There are efforts underway that attempt to bridge social factors with care delivery. Community health worker interventions represent an effort to bridge communities and health care systems. The VA implementation of a network of community based outpatient clinics represents an effort to connect care access for Veterans in less-populated areas. It is important to consider not only disparities that may arise from clinician biases and organizational deficiencies in cultural competence, but also to incorporate an understanding of patient circumstances in their lived environment. Accounting for what transpires for Veterans as they move from clinician offices through their communities and into their homes may expand the possibilities for reducing and eliminating disparities in care and outcomes.

Figure 2 details our conceptual mapping of areas bearing influence on health outcomes for individuals, which span from the patient-provider interaction to the environments where individuals live and work. In addition, figure 2 describe our meta-findings by mapping interventions identified in this review that bridge areas where disparities in health care and outcomes arise. By considering the entire spectrum, we are able to identify potential for intervention strategies to expand the reach of health systems. While specific interventions tackling disparities arising from particular nodes are associated with limited or equivocal evidence (i.e., clinical reminders), more effective interventions reach beyond one limited area to address multiple components simultaneously (i.e., case management, community health workers, tailored health education). Conceptually, these interventions are more successful at addressing disparities that emerge and operate at different levels. This conceptual diagram also demonstrates the importance of incorporating social factors into the discussion of addressing disparities in health outcomes. In the future, studies designed to address race/ethnic disparities in health should be explicit about where interventions fall within these conceptual ellipses. Based on our review, interventions that span across multiple ellipses may prove to be more effective than more limited interventions.

The strength of interventions lies in the connectedness of intervention programs to the individuals they are meant to reach, as well as the consideration of underlying patient health needs and socioeconomic means. The diagram acknowledges that the effectiveness of interventions that span across providers, health care systems, neighborhood environments and individual residences are at least partly dependent on patient demographics (e.g., age, gender, literacy), individual socioeconomic means and neighborhood structural qualities (e.g., safe and abundant places to exercise) and health needs (e.g. severe chronic conditions). Based on this review, interventions that include comprehensive care management efforts, evidence-based health education programs, and consistent, well-trained community health workers show potential for reducing disparities in health and health care for minority Veterans.

Figure 2. Conceptual Model—Reach of Interventions

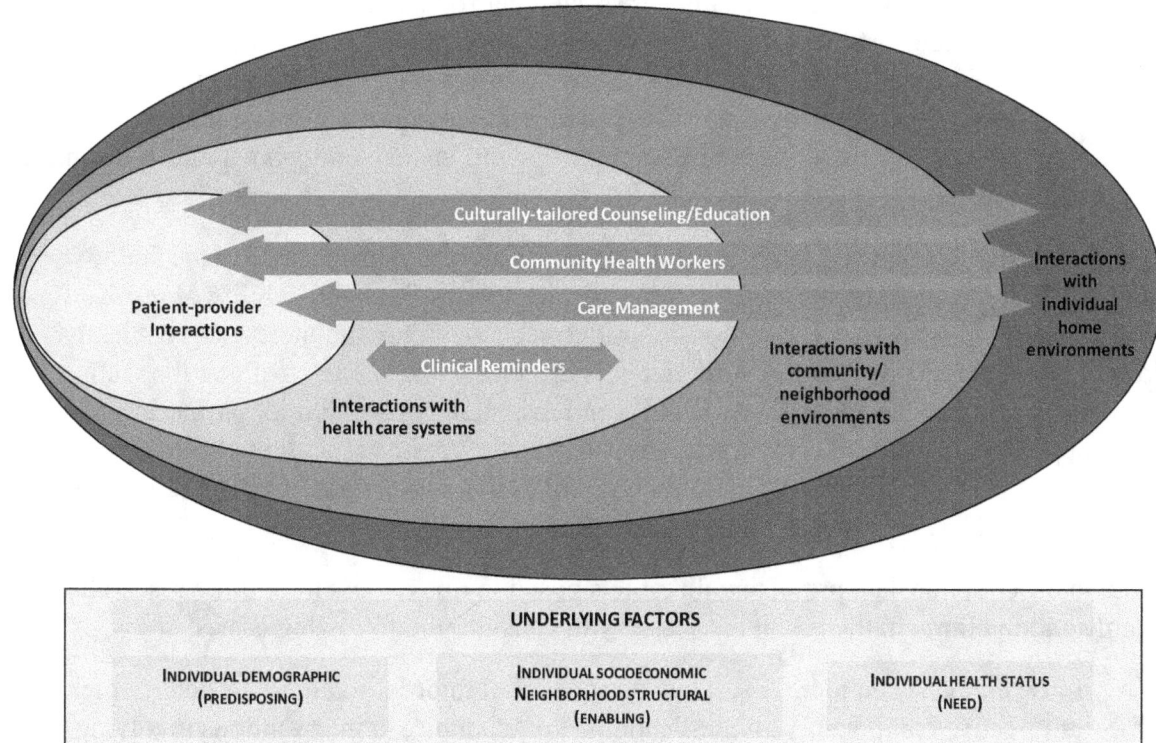

FUTURE RESEARCH AND IMPLICATIONS FOR VA HEALTH CARE SETTINGS

There are several key steps that may aid in the development, testing, and implementation of disparities interventions that could help fill some of the many identified evidence gaps. First and foremost, continuing the VA policy to consistently collect race and ethnicity information for all Veterans is to be encouraged. The ongoing concerted effort to populate race/ethnicity in the VA data records is a critical step to chronicling progress in reducing disparities for minority Veterans.

Capacity assessment also forms an important precondition with regard to intervention implementation in the VA. Two active war theaters imply changes in the Veteran population that will result in near-term burdens on the VA health care system. Efforts to improve knowledge and expertise of providers (e.g., through cultural competence training) will increase awareness of disparities in care and outcomes among minority Veterans.

In addition, there are practical and operational considerations to implementing promising interventions. For example, the use of community health workers was frequently identified as a strategy that holds promise for reaching minority populations. However there is substantial heterogeneity in the composition, training, monitoring, frequency of contact and setting for peer health workers. Identifying optimal characteristics (e.g., training protocols, forms, software) for these interventions is necessary for effective implementation. Documentation and implementation details (including unanticipated challenges and solutions) should be encouraged.

A recent study of VA health care trends found that, although gaps in process measures between black and white Veterans in the VA health care system narrowed after the implementation of quality improvement efforts, significant differences in clinical outcomes have persisted, most notably in heart disease, diabetes and hypertension.[54] Most studies included in our review focused on process of care outcomes and few examine the effects on distal health outcomes. Future studies should sustain longer follow-up periods and include enough patients to examine distal health outcomes.

The vast majority of reviewed interventions also relied on results from small-scale study settings with limited geographic scope. This raises questions of generalizability of results, and VA capacity for scaling these demonstration projects to larger and more geographically representative Veteran populations. Although it is difficult – and risky – to argue for scaling up promising pilot studies of small-scale interventions, there is potential for partnering with already-deployed, large, multicenter programs such as the VA's patient aligned care team (PACT) demonstration projects. In this way, multiple initiatives that require access to a large pool of Veterans can be addressed with a single research investment.

In sum, in order to translate promising directions posed in this review into future research and implementation efforts in the VA, it is necessary to consider the following issues:

- Interventions need to be described in more detail in order to allow for determination of effective components of interventions. For example, in interventions involving community health workers and care managers, there was poor specification of the training of those personnel.
- Integrate the use of community health workers into VA settings. This could involve Veteran peer advisors coming from communities where Veterans reside.
- Examine the potential for ongoing, large VA demonstration projects in care coordination/care management to improve the health of minority Veterans and reduce disparities.
- Enhance the capacity to tailor patient educational materials to address the specific needs of minority Veterans.
- Consider funding studies explicitly designed to measure pre-post changes in disparities between minority and white Veterans.
- Encourage the inclusion of less well studied minority Veteran groups (i.e., Asian/Pacific Islander and American Indian) in the design and implementation of disparities studies.

There are also opportunities for studies conducted in single VAMCs – such as the lessons offered by the five included primary VA research studies – to provide important discussion of how to best reduce disparities for minority Veterans. Future third generation research specific to VAMCs should be encouraged and disseminated in order for VA researchers and implementers to benefit from a robust evidence base. From a practical standpoint, there is room for "disparities teams" at individual VAMCs to learn from collective knowledge gained across various VA sites. Sharing lessons and promising strategies for reducing disparities from ongoing research projects through periodic communication between disparities interest groups may serve to quicken dissemination of actionable results to VA equity stakeholders.

Given the low yield of VA intervention studies identified in our search of published literature, we examined the abstracts of recently funded HSR&D studies to determine whether intervention studies for racial/ethnic disparities are in progress. We reviewed 89 titles and abstracts of projects in the HSR&D Equity Portfolio and found four projects containing race-specific interventions: Improving Dental Decision Making for Root Canal Therapy (Kressin N), Tailoring Coping Skills Training for African Americans with Osteoarthritis (Allen K), Knee Replacement Disparity: A Randomized, Controlled Intervention (Ibrahim S), Proactive Tobacco Treatment for Diverse Veteran Smokers (Fu S). There were three career development awardees with potentially relevant project titles, although the details of study design are not currently available: Understanding & Reducing Racial Disparities in Renal Transplantation (Myaskovsky L), Understanding & Ameliorating Racial/Ethnic Disparities in Healthcare (Burgess D), Identifying Mechanisms Linking Perceived Discrimination & Health (Hausmann, L).

Few disparities interventions have been implemented in the VA, and although a few race-specific intervention studies are underway, much more work is needed in this area. The barriers to implementing disparities intervention research in VA care settings are not entirely clear. Future steps emanating from this review will include conducting a survey and interviews of key VA informants to identify barriers to dissemination of interventions, in an effort to provide a better understanding of the obstructions in the VA disparities research pipeline.

REFERENCES

1. Chang C, Jackson SS, Bullman TA, Cobbs EL. Impact of a home-based primary care program in an urban Veterans Affairs medical center. *J Am Med Dir Assoc.* Feb 2009;10(2):133-137.

2. Dang S, Remon N, Harris J, et al. Care coordination assisted by technology for multiethnic caregivers of persons with dementia: a pilot clinical demonstration project on caregiver burden and depression. *J Telemed Telecare.* 2008;14(8):443-447.

3. Shore JH, Brooks E, Savin D, Orton H, Grigsby J, Manson SM. Acceptability of telepsychiatry in American Indians. *Telemed J E Health.* Jun 2008;14(5):461-466.

4. Dang S, Ma F, Nedd N, Florez H, Aguilar E, Roos BA. Care coordination and telemedicine improves glycaemic control in ethnically diverse veterans with diabetes. *J Telemed Telecare.* 2007;13(5):263-267.

5. Weng HH, Kaplan RM, Boscardin WJ, et al. Development of a decision aid to address racial disparities in utilization of knee replacement surgery. *Arthritis Rheum.* May 15 2007;57(4):568-575.

6. Hawthorne K, Robles Y, Cannings-John R, Edwards AG. Culturally appropriate health education for Type 2 diabetes in ethnic minority groups: a systematic and narrative review of randomized controlled trials. *Diabet Med.* Jun 2010;27(6):613-623.

7. Hawthorne K, Robles Y, Cannings-John R, Edwards AG. Culturally appropriate health education for type 2 diabetes mellitus in ethnic minority groups. *Cochrane Database Syst Rev.* 2008(3):CD006424.

8. Peek ME, Cargill A, Huang ES. Diabetes health disparities: a systematic review of health care interventions. *Med Care Res Rev.* Oct 2007;64(5 Suppl):101S-156S.

9. Saxena S, Misra T, Car J, Netuveli G, Smith R, Majeed A. Systematic review of primary healthcare interventions to improve diabetes outcomes in minority ethnic groups. *J Ambul Care Manage.* Jul-Sep 2007;30(3):218-230.

10. Norris SL, Chowdhury FM, Van Le K, et al. Effectiveness of community health workers in the care of persons with diabetes. *Diabet Med.* May 2006;23(5):544-556.

11. Sarkisian CA, Brown AF, Norris KC, Wintz RL, Mangione CM. A systematic review of diabetes self-care interventions for older, African American, or Latino adults. *Diabetes Educ.* May-Jun 2003;29(3):467-479.

12. McIlvane JM, Baker TA, Mingo CA, Haley WE. Are behavioral interventions for arthritis effective with minorities? Addressing racial and ethnic diversity in disability and rehabilitation. *Arthritis Rheum.* Oct 15 2008;59(10):1512-1518.

13. Ettinger WH, Jr., Burns R, Messier SP, et al. A randomized trial comparing aerobic exercise and resistance exercise with a health education program in older adults with knee osteoarthritis. The Fitness Arthritis and Seniors Trial (FAST). *JAMA*. Jan 1 1997;277(1):25-31.

14. Penninx BW, Messier SP, Rejeski WJ, et al. Physical exercise and the prevention of disability in activities of daily living in older persons with osteoarthritis. *Archives of Internal Medicine*. Oct 22 2001;161(19):2309-2316.

15. Corcoran J, Dattalo P, Crowley M. Interventions to increase mammography rates among U.S. Latinas: a systematic review. *J Womens Health (Larchmt)*. Jul 2010;19(7):1281-1288.

16. Martinez-Donate AP. Using lay health advisors to promote breast and cervical cancer screening among Latinas: a review. *WMJ*. Aug 2009;108(5):259-262.

17. Han HR, Lee JE, Kim J, Hedlin HK, Song H, Kim MT. A meta-analysis of interventions to promote mammography among ethnic minority women. *Nurs Res*. Jul-Aug 2009;58(4):246-254.

18. Masi CM, Blackman DJ, Peek ME. Interventions to enhance breast cancer screening, diagnosis, and treatment among racial and ethnic minority women. *Med Care Res Rev*. Oct 2007;64(5 Suppl):195S-242S.

19. O'Malley AS, Gonzalez RM, Sheppard VB, Huerta E, Mandelblatt J. Primary care cancer control interventions including Latinos: a review. *Am J Prev Med*. Oct 2003;25(3):264-271.

20. Han HR, Kim J, Lee JE, et al. Interventions that increase use of Pap tests among ethnic minority women: a meta-analysis. *Psychooncology*. Apr 29 2010.

21. Powe BD, Faulkenberry R, Harmond L. A review of intervention studies that seek to increase colorectal cancer screening among African-Americans. *Am J Health Promot*. Nov-Dec 2010;25(2):92-99.

22. Morrow JB, Dallo FJ, Julka M. Community-Based Colorectal Cancer Screening Trials with Multi-Ethnic Groups: A Systematic Review. *J Community Health*. Mar 12 2010.

23. Webb MS. Treating tobacco dependence among African Americans: a meta-analytic review. *Health Psychol*. May 2008;27(3 Suppl):S271-282.

24. Webb MS, Rodriguez-Esquivel D, Baker EA. Smoking cessation interventions among Hispanics in the United States: A systematic review and mini meta-analysis. *Am J Health Promot*. Nov-Dec 2010;25(2):109-118.

25. Davis AM, Vinci LM, Okwuosa TM, Chase AR, Huang ES. Cardiovascular health disparities: a systematic review of health care interventions. *Med Care Res Rev*. Oct 2007;64(5 Suppl):29S-100S.

26. Whitt-Glover MC, Kumanyika SK. Systematic review of interventions to increase physical activity and physical fitness in African-Americans. *Am J Health Promot.* Jul-Aug 2009;23(6):S33-56.

27. Osei-Assibey G, Kyrou I, Adi Y, Kumar S, Matyka K. Dietary and lifestyle interventions for weight management in adults from minority ethnic/non-White groups: a systematic review. *Obes Rev.* Jan 6 2010.

28. Eyles HC, Mhurchu CN. Does tailoring make a difference? A systematic review of the long-term effectiveness of tailored nutrition education for adults. *Nutr Rev.* Aug 2009;67(8):464-480.

29. Perez-Escamilla R, Hromi-Fiedler A, Vega-Lopez S, Bermudez-Millan A, Segura-Perez S. Impact of peer nutrition education on dietary behaviors and health outcomes among Latinos: a systematic literature review. *J Nutr Educ Behav.* Jul-Aug 2008;40(4):208-225.

30. Crook ED, Bryan NB, Hanks R, et al. A review of interventions to reduce health disparities in cardiovascular disease in African Americans. *Ethn Dis.* Spring 2009;19(2):204-208.

31. Mau MK, Sinclair K, Saito EP, Baumhofer KN, Kaholokula JK. Cardiometabolic health disparities in native Hawaiians and other Pacific Islanders. *Epidemiol Rev.* 2009;31:113-129.

32. Crepaz N, Marshall KJ, Aupont LW, et al. The efficacy of HIV/STI behavioral interventions for African American females in the United States: a meta-analysis. *Am J Public Health.* Nov 2009;99(11):2069-2078.

33. Crepaz N, Horn AK, Rama SM, et al. The efficacy of behavioral interventions in reducing HIV risk sex behaviors and incident sexually transmitted disease in black and Hispanic sexually transmitted disease clinic patients in the United States: a meta-analytic review. *Sex Transm Dis.* Jun 2007;34(6):319-332.

34. Johnson BT, Scott-Sheldon LA, Smoak ND, Lacroix JM, Anderson JR, Carey MP. Behavioral interventions for African Americans to reduce sexual risk of HIV: a meta-analysis of randomized controlled trials. *J Acquir Immune Defic Syndr.* Aug 1 2009;51(4):492-501.

35. Herbst JH, Kay LS, Passin WF, et al. A systematic review and meta-analysis of behavioral interventions to reduce HIV risk behaviors of Hispanics in the United States and Puerto Rico. *AIDS Behav.* Jan 2007;11(1):25-47.

36. Van Voorhees BW, Walters AE, Prochaska M, Quinn MT. Reducing health disparities in depressive disorders outcomes between non-Hispanic Whites and ethnic minorities: a call for pragmatic strategies over the life course. *Med Care Res Rev.* Oct 2007;64(5 Suppl):157S-194S.

37. Ward EC. Examining differential treatment effects for depression in racial and ethnic minority women: a qualitative systematic review. *J Natl Med Assoc.* Mar 2007;99(3):265-274.

38. Lie DA, Lee-Rey E, Gomez A, Bereknyei S, Braddock CH, 3rd. Does Cultural Competency Training of Health Professionals Improve Patient Outcomes? A Systematic Review and Proposed Algorithm for Future Research. *J Gen Intern Med.* Oct 16 2010.

39. Bhui K, Warfa N, Edonya P, McKenzie K, Bhugra D. Cultural competence in mental health care: a review of model evaluations. *BMC Health Serv Res.* 2007;7:15.

40. Beach MC, Gary TL, Price EG, et al. Improving health care quality for racial/ethnic minorities: a systematic review of the best evidence regarding provider and organization interventions. *BMC Public Health.* 2006;6:104.

41. Beach MC, Price EG, Gary TL, et al. Cultural competence: a systematic review of health care provider educational interventions. *Med Care.* Apr 2005;43(4):356-373.

42. Anderson LM, Scrimshaw SC, Fullilove MT, Fielding JE, Normand J, Task Force on Community Preventive S. Culturally competent healthcare systems. A systematic review. *Am J Prev Med.* Apr 2003;24(3 Suppl):68-79.

43. Perry E, Swartz J, Brown S, et al. Peer mentoring: a culturally sensitive approach to end-of-life planning for long-term dialysis patients. *American Journal of Kidney Diseases.* Jul 2005;46(1):111-119.

44. Sequist TD, Fitzmaurice GM, Marshall R, et al. Cultural competency training and performance reports to improve diabetes care for black patients: a cluster randomized, controlled trial. *Annals of Internal Medicine.* Jan 5 2010;152(1):40-46.

45. Kilbourne AM, Switzer G, Hyman K, et al. Advancing health disparities research within the health care system: a conceptual framework. *American Journal of Public Health.* Dec 2006;96(12):2113-2121.

46. Fine MJ, Ibrahim SA, Thomas SB, Fine MJ, Ibrahim SA, Thomas SB. The role of race and genetics in health disparities research. *American Journal of Public Health.* Dec 2005;95(12):2125-2128.

47. Wong MD, Shapiro MF, Boscardin WJ, et al. Contribution of major diseases to disparities in mortality. *New England Journal of Medicine.* Nov 14 2002;347(20):1585-1592.

48. Cooper R, Cutler J, Desvigne-Nickens P, et al. Trends and disparities in coronary heart disease, stroke, and other cardiovascular diseases in the United States: findings of the national conference on cardiovascular disease prevention. *Circulation.* Dec 19 2000;102(25):3137-3147.

49. Hayward M, Miles T, Crimmins E, Yang Y. The significance of socioeconomic status in explaining the racial gap in chronic health conditions. *American Sociological Review.* 2000;65(6):910-930.

50. Saha S, Freeman M, Toure J, Tippens KM, Weeks C, Ibrahim S. Racial and ethnic disparities in the VA health care system: a systematic review. *J Gen Intern Med.* May 2008;23(5):654-671.

51. Gehlert S, Sohmer D, Sacks T, et al. Targeting health disparities: a model linking upstream determinants to downstream interventions. *Health Affairs.* Mar-Apr 2008;27(2):339-349.

52. Gruen RL, Pearson SD, Brennan TA, Gruen RL, Pearson SD, Brennan TA. Physician-citizens--public roles and professional obligations. *JAMA.* Jan 7 2004;291(1):94-98.

53. Thomas S, Crouse Q, Butler J, Fryer C, Garza M. Toward a fourth generation of disparities research to acheive health equity. *Annual Review of Public Health.* 2011;32:309-416.

54. Trivedi A, Grebla R, Wright S, Washington D. Despite improved quality of care in the Veterans Affairs health system, racial disparity persists for important clinical outcomes. *Health Affairs.* 2011;30(4):707-715.

APPENDIX A. SEARCH STRATEGY

I. SEARCH FOR INTERVENTION STUDIES TO REDUCE RACIAL DISPARITIES

Search	Most Recent Queries	Time	Result
#12	Search systematic[sb] AND (#9)	15:47:12	2129
#9	Search (#8) OR #6	15:43:46	83980
#8	Search (#4) AND #7	15:43:29	25879
#7	Search "Evaluation Studies "[Publication Type] OR "Clinical Trial "[Publication Type]	15:43:08	751037
#6	Search (#5) AND #4	15:42:49	65155
#5	Search address OR program OR intervention* OR reduce OR eliminate[Title/Abstract]	15:42:38	1106596
#4	Search ((#3) OR #2) OR #1	15:42:29	491858
#3	Search (("Population Groups"[Mesh] OR "Race Relations"[Mesh]) OR "Minority Groups"[Mesh]) OR "Health Services Accessibility"[Mesh]	15:41:47	229846
#2	Search ethnic* OR race or Racial OR disparity OR disparities OR blacks OR black OR hispanic* OR equity OR sociodemographic OR discrimination OR minority OR minorities OR "African american*"[Title/Abstract]	15:41:36	425423
#1	Search (((("African Continental Ancestry Group"[Mesh] OR "Hispanic Americans"[Mesh]) OR "Indians, North American"[Mesh]) OR "Inuits"[Mesh]) OR "Asian Americans"[Mesh]	15:41:16	77830

II. UPDATE SEARCH FOR RECENTLY PUBLISHED STUDIES USING THE STRATEGY DESIGNED FOR THE 2007 VA- ESP REVIEW OF PRIMARY VA STUDIES

Search terms in PubMed Database Searched August 12, 2010

((VA [tw] OR veteran* [tw]) OR (United States Department of Veterans Affairs [mh] OR veterans [mh] OR veterans hospitals [mh])) AND ((ethnic* [tw] OR race [tw] OR racial [tw] OR disparity [tw] OR disparities [tw] OR blacks [tw] OR black [tw] OR Hispanic* [tw]) OR (population groups [mh] OR race relations [mh])) AND (("2006/10/01"[PDat] : "3000"[PDat]))

Result: 533

Search terms in HSRProj Database Searched August 12, 2010

VA and (disparity OR disparities OR equity)
and Project Status = Ongoing & Completed (Default)
and Initial Year from: 2006 To: 2010
States: All

Result: 31 Projects

III. Search for systematic reviews of intervention studies on racial disparities

Search	Most Recent Queries
#12	Search **systematic[sb] AND (#9)**
#9	Search **(#8) OR #6**
#8	Search **(#4) AND #7**
#7	Search **"Evaluation Studies "[Publication Type] OR "Clinical Trial "[Publication Type]**
#6	Search **(#5) AND #4**
#5	Search **address OR program OR intervention* OR reduce OR eliminate[Title/Abstract]**
#4	Search **((#3) OR #2) OR #1**
#3	Search **(("Population Groups"[Mesh] OR "Race Relations"[Mesh]) OR "Minority Groups"[Mesh]) OR "Health Services Accessibility"[Mesh]**
#2	Search **ethnic* OR race or Racial OR disparity OR disparities OR blacks OR black OR hispanic* OR equity OR sociodemographic OR discrimination OR minority OR minorities OR "African american*"[Title/Abstract]**
#1	Search **(((("African Continental Ancestry Group"[Mesh] OR "Hispanic Americans"[Mesh]) OR "Indians, North American"[Mesh]) OR "Inuits"[Mesh]) OR "Asian Americans"[Mesh]**

APPENDIX B. INCLUSION/EXCLUSION CRITERIA FOR PRIMARY STUDIES AND REVIEWS

1. Is the full text of the article in English?
   Yes ....Proceed to #2
   No ....Code **X1**. Go to #6

2. Does the study population include adults in the U.S.?
   Yes ....Proceed to #3
   No ....Code **X2**. Go to #6

3. Does the article evaluate the effects of an intervention within one or more racial/ethnic minority group(s), or between racial/ethnic groups including at least one racial/ethnic minority group?
   Yes ....Proceed to #4
   No ....Code **X3**. Go to #6

4. Is the publication a primary study conducted in a VA population, or a systematic review or meta-analysis (not limited to VA) that meets methodological quality criteria?
   Yes ....Proceed to #5
   No ....Code X4. Proceed to #6

5. Is the intervention applicable to VA care settings?
   (Applicability refers to patient populations and disease entities of documented disparities in the VA setting. Qualifying interventions must target services provided at the VA. Obstetric care and interventions designed to improve access are examples of exclusions)
   Yes ....Code I5. STOP
   No ....Code X5. Proceed to #6

6. Is the article potentially useful for background, discussion, or reference-mining?
   Yes ....Add code B. STOP
   No ....STOP

> *PICOTS*
>
> *Population*: adults in the US. Studies exclusively on children or adolescents are excluded.
>
> *Interventions:* third generation studies that evaluate the effects of an intervention within one or more racial/ethnic minority group(s) or between racial/ethnic groups including at least one racial/ethnic minority group.
>
> *Comparator:* control group within same racial/ethnic minority group, or comparison between racial/ethnic groups.
>
> *Outcomes:* not limited. outcomes of interest include the following:
>
>   i. Utilization of health care services
>   ii. Quality of health care services
>   1. Process of care measures (e.g., use of appropriate screening tests)
>   2. Outcome measures used by VHA as quality metrics (e.g., blood pressure control)
>   3. Patient evaluations of care (e.g., patient satisfaction)
>   4. Direct observations of care (e.g., communication patterns)
>   iii. Potential mediators of racial/ethnic disparities in utilization or quality
>   1. System-level mediators (e.g., distribution of services)
>   2. Provider-level mediators (e.g., racial bias)
>   3. Patient-level mediators (e.g., trust)
>   iv. Patient-provider level mediators (e.g., communication)
>   v. Health outcomes (e.g., diabetic complications)
>
> *Timing:* any length of followup
>
> *Setting:* US

APPENDIX C. QUALITY RATING CRITERIA FOR REVIEWS

Overall quality rating for systematic reviews is based on the questions below. Ratings are summarized as: *Good, Fair, or Poor*:*

- Search dates reported? *Yes or No*
- Search methods reported? *Yes or No*
- Comprehensive search? *Yes or No*
- Inclusion criteria reported? *Yes or No*
- Selection bias avoided? *Yes or No*
- Validity criteria reported? *Yes or No*
- Validity assessed appropriately? *Yes or No*
- Methods used to combine studies reported? *Yes or No*
- Findings combined appropriately? *Yes or No*
- Conclusions supported by data? *Yes or No*

Definitions of ratings based on above criteria

Good: Meet all criteria: Reports comprehensive and reproducible search methods and results; reports pre-defined criteria to select studies and reports reasons for excluding potentially relevant studies; adequately evaluates quality of included studies and incorporates assessments of quality when synthesizing data; reports methods for synthesizing data and uses appropriate methods to combine data qualitatively or quantitatively; conclusions supported by the evidence reviewed.

Fair: Studies will be graded fair if they fail to meet one or more of the above criteria, but the limitations are not judged as being major.

Poor: Studies will be graded poor if they have a major limitation in one or more of the above criteria.

*Created from the following publications:

Harris RP, Helfand M, Woolf SH, et al. Current methods of the US Preventive Services Task Force: a review of the process. *Am J Prev Med.* 2001:20(3S); 21-35.

National Institute for Health and Clinical Excellence. The Guidelines Manual. London: Institute for Health and Clinical Excellence; 2006.

Oxman AD, Guyatt GH. Validation of an index of the quality of review articles. *J Clin Epidemiol.* 1991;44:1271-8.

APPENDIX D. EVIDENCE TABLE

Author, Year, EN ID	Clinical topic	Population	Setting	Single-race (included only minority study participants)	Comparative (included minority and majority participants with pre and post intervention comparison)	Mostly generic or tailored interventions?	Study methodology (e.g., systematic review, meta-analysis)	Study period/search dates	Number and hierarchy of studies included	Intervention types (i.e., community health workers)
Primary Studies										
Chang, 2009[1]	Preventive	Veterans n=183 patients 71% black, 29% white	Urban VAMC (Washington DC)	No	Yes. Multiple groups, but do not analyze pre-post by race	Generic	Primary article; retrospective chart review of HBPC enrollees. Pre-post enrollment (no control)	Patients enrolled for at least 6 months during the period of January 2001-December 2002	n/a	Multiprofessional home-based primary care (HBPC) team: medical director, nurse practitioners, registered nurses, social workers, pharmacists, registered dietician, dental hygienist and program director.
Dang, 2007[4]	Preventive	Veterans age 60 or older n=41 patients n=21 white (51%) n=14 black (34%) n=6 Hispanic (15%)	Urban VAMC (Miami)	No	Yes	Generic	Primary study (pre-post no control group)	Patients enrolled for at least 9 months from May 2000-January 2002	n/a	Care coordination: 2 care coordinators (nurse pract, licensed clin social worker), secretary and geriatrician (oversight) Telemedicine: telephone-based in-home messaging device for patient monitoring. Patients input blood sugar levels and answer educational questions. Data transmitted to messaging center, stratified into high/med/low risk for care coordinators following morning.
Dang, 2008[2]	Mental health	Veterans with dementia (MMSE < 25) and live-in caregivers; white = 72, AA = 32, Hispanic = 9.	Homes of caregivers/recipients.	No	Yes. Multiple groups, but do not analyze pre-post by race	Generic	Primary article; pre-post with no control group	n/a	n/a	Screen telephones and support by care coordinators.
Shore, 2008[3]	Mental health	American Indian Vietnam Veterans	In person and telephone interviews	Yes	No	Tailored	Primary article; tests of mean differences, comparisons of kappas.	n/a	n/a	Telephone and in person interviews to test the feasibility of SCID in this population/setting
Weng, 2007[5]	Pain/arthritis	African American and white male Veterans n=102 patients at baseline (n=54 black and n=48 white) n=64 completed followup questionnaire (n=33 black, n=31 white)	Urban VAMC (Greater Los Angeles)	No	Yes	Tailored	Primary study (pre-post no control group)	n/a	n/a	Educational videotape and tailored total knee replacement (TKR) decision aid
Systematic Reviews										
Anderson, 2003[40]	Cross-cutting	Minorities only	All medical settings	Yes. Most included studies are single-race.	No	Tailored	Systematic review	1965-2001	6 RCTs	Clinician bias: recruitment/retention of diverse staff, interpreter services, cultural competence training, ed materials, culturally specific health care settings.
Beach, 2005[39]	Cross-cutting	Health professionals and ethnic minority patients	n/a	Yes. Most included studies are single-race.	No	Tailored	Systematic review	1980 through 2/2003	2 RCTs, 12 controlled, 20 pre-post.	Training programs varying in lengths generally effective in improving certain aspects of provider characteristics.
Beach, 2006[38]	Preventive	Physicians, nurses and medical assistants and emergency medical personnel.	Hospital outpatient Community health center Group practice Community care	Yes. Some included studies are single-race.	Yes. Most included studies are comparative.	Tailored	Systematic review	1980-June 2003	n=27 RCT n=20 CCT n=7	Tracking/reminder systems, bypassing the physician, safe times questionnaires for pts, remote simultaneous translation

Interventions to Improve Minority Health Care and Reduce Racial and Ethnic Disparities

Evidence-based Synthesis Program

Author, Year, EN ID	Clinical topic	Population	Setting	Single-race (included only minority study participants)	Comparative (included minority and majority participants with pre and post intervention comparison)	Mostly generic or tailored interventions?	Study methodology (e.g., systematic review, meta-analysis)	Study period/search dates	Number and hierarchy of studies included	Intervention types (i.e., community health workers)
Corcoran, 2010[13]	Preventive	Latinas in the US	Community (6) and clinic (3) settings in California, Texas, New Mexico, Colorado and Washington	Yes. All included studies are single-race.	No	Tailored	Meta-analysis	ended January 2009	n=9 Quasi-experimental n=6 RCT n=3	Lay-health advisor (promotoras), printed mailings, educational groups, television campaigns, access-enhancing (1 study)
Crepaz, 2007[31]	HIV/AIDS	Black and Hispanic STD Clinic Patients	STD Clinics	No	Yes. Some included studies are comparative, but do not analyze pre-post by race.	Tailored	Meta-analysis	1998-june 2005	18 RCTs	Intervention delivered by health educator/counselor
Crepaz, 2009[30]	HIV/AIDS	African American Females	Health Care and Community Settings	Yes	Yes. Some included studies are comparative, but do not analyze pre-post by race.	Tailored	Meta-analysis	January 1988 to June 2007	37 individual and groups level intervention studies and 4 community level intervention studies.	Patient activation
Crook, 2009[28]	CVD	African-Americans	Ambulatory care and community settings	Yes	No	Generic	Systematic review	1996 - 2006	NR	Counseling/education for behavior change; screening; changes in delivery system; exercise, stress reduction, dietary modification
Davis, 2007[27]	CVD	Minorities and whites	Community and health care settings. Interventions had to be connected to health care organizations.	Yes. Most included studies are single-race.	Yes. Some included studies are comparative, but do not analyze pre-post by race.	Generic	Systematic review	1995 - 2006	Overall: 52 RCT, 8 pre-post, 2 non-randomized controlled clinical trials	Provider and care delivery interventions (e.g., patient outreach, clinic reorganization, interventions with nurses alone or with community health workers included); patient and family interventions
Eyles, 2009[25]	Preventive	Health or mixed-health status adults aged 18 to 85+	Non-face-to-face methods of contacting participants. Of the US studies, 6 were conducted in community settings, 4 were conducted in clinical/health care settings and 2 did not report recruitment activities.	Yes. One included study was single-race.	Yes	Tailored	Meta-analysis (and narrative summaries)	January 1990-December 2007	n=16 All studies were RCT or quasi-RCT All studies included experimental group that received tailored nutrition education and control group with either generic and/or no nutrition education. 11 were conducted in the US, 1 was conducted in US and Canada	Tailored nutrition education included print, email or other non-face-to-face format (excluded studies that used face-to-face delivery methods)
Han, 2009[15]	Preventive	Adult Asian/PI, African American, Hispanic and white women	n=19 in community settings n=4 in health care settings	Yes. Most included studies are single-race.	Yes. Some included studies are comparative, but do not analyze pre-post by race.	Tailored	Meta-analysis	September 2000 - August 2008	n=23 RCT n=14 All studies were experimental or quasi-experimental design. Evidence tables offered as supplemental online content	directed print materials, peer/lay health advisor education and support, telephone counseling.
Han, 2010[18]	Preventive	Adult women. N=4 predominantly African American; N=3 mostly Hispanic; N=8 mostly Asian; N=1 mostly Native American; N=2 combination of Hispanic and African American	n=5 health care settings n=13 community settings	Yes. Most included studies are single-race.	Yes	Generic	Meta-analysis	1984-April 2009	n=18 RCT n=9 Quasi-experimental non randomized n=9	1. Individual-directed (in-person and phone counseling) 2. Access-enhancing (reduced cost, mobile vans) 3. Peer-navigator (lay health advisors) 4. Community education (small group workshops/seminars) 5. Mass media (tv, newspaper, radio campaigns)

Interventions to Improve Minority Health Care and Reduce Racial and Ethnic Disparities

Author, Year, EN ID	Clinical topic	Population	Setting	Single-race (included only minority study participants)	Comparative (included minority and majority participants with pre and post intervention comparison)	Mostly generic or tailored interventions?	Study methodology (e.g., systematic review, meta-analysis)	Study period/search dates	Number and hierarchy of studies included	Intervention types (i.e.: community health workers)
Hawthorne, 2010[6] Hawthorne 2008[7]	Diabetes	All included studies were conducted in single-race groups. Some populations don't apply to US (e.g. South Asian British).	Group and individual sessions in clinics, community medical centers, homes of participants, hospital and GP practices. Type of HE provider ranged from peer leaders, certified DM educators, bilingual nurse, CHW, podiatrist, dietician, exercise physiotherapist.	Yes. All included studies were conducted in single-race groups.	No	Tailored	Systematic review and meta-analysis	1966 or inception thru 2007	12 RCTs	Culturally appropriate health education (group sessions in the majority of included studies) defined as HE tailored to the cultural or religious beliefs and linguistic and literacy skills of the community being studied.
Herbst, 2007[33]	HIV/AIDS	Hispanics	Health/drug treatment clinics, schools, community based organizations, and farm worker campsites	Yes	No	Tailored	Meta-analysis	1988-2006	20 studies included in meta-analysis	Variety of implementation methods from fotonovela to health educator/outreach worker
Johnson, 2009[32]	HIV/AIDS	African Americans	Community and clinical settings	Yes	Yes. Most included studies are comparative, but do not analyze pre-post by race.	Tailored	Meta-analysis	1981-2006	78 RCTs	Health education
Lie, 2010[36]	Cross-cutting	All patient populations	All medical settings	Yes. One included study was single-race.	No	Tailored	Systematic review	1/1990-3/2010	2 quasi-randomized, 2 cluster randomized, 3 pre-post.	Cultural competence curricula
Martinez-Donate, 2009[14]	Preventive	Latinas and non-Latinas in the US	Community setting; majority of included studies in the West and Southwest US	No	Yes	Generic	Systematic review	Through August 2008	N=14 RCT N=2 CCT N=6	Lay health advisors (education, phone counseling, media campaign, social support, community events, mobile screening)
Masi, 2007[16]	Preventive	Minority and white female patients (mostly African American and Hispanic); providers	Health care settings	Yes. A few included studies are single-race.	Yes. Most included studies are comparative.	Generic	Systematic review	1986-December 2005	n=43 (n=36 on screening, n=5 follow up testing, n=2 treatment, n=1 survivorship) RCT n=33 CCT=10	Patient: reminder letters, telephone calls, written educational materials, in-person counseling, mammography vouchers, classroom education Provider: chart reminders, chart flow sheets, written education materials, chart autids with feedback
Mau, 2009[29]	CVD	Native Hawaiians and other Pacific Islanders (NHOPI)	2 community based samples, 1 clinic sample	Yes	No	Tailored	Systematic review	1998 - 2008	2 pre-post, 1 nonrandomized controlled clinical trial	One study used community health workers to deliver a disease management program. Another study used group visits for hypertension counseling.
Morrow, 2010[20]	Preventive	Multiethnic groups in the US, including at least 1 disadvantaged group	Community-based	No	Yes	Generic	Systematic review	1/2001 - 8/2009	N=15 All RCT	1. Patient mailings (mailing, tailored mailing & phone reminder, brochure); N=3 2. Telephone outreach (scripted and unscripted phone assistance with mailings, care manager calls, tailored phone education); N=3 3. Electronic and multimedia (physician email system, preferences-based website, standardized website, multimedia computer program education, peer education/health professional video education); N=4 4. Community education (pts receiving navigator services, community screening behavior program, risk counseling, general counseling, cultural self-empowerment) N=5
Ngo-Metzger, 2010[53]	Cross-cutting	Asian American patients, though NO articles were found on this population.	All medical settings	Yes	No	Generic	Systematic review	1/1994-7/2009	None. Extrapolate from white patients.	Some recommendations at end, none based on any evidence.

Evidence-based Synthesis Program

46

Interventions to Improve Minority Health Care and Reduce Racial and Ethnic Disparities

Author, Year, EN ID	Clinical topic	Population	Setting	Single-race (included only minority study participants)	Comparative (included minority and majority participants with pre and post intervention comparison)	Mostly generic or tailored interventions?	Study methodology (e.g., systematic review, meta-analysis)	Study period/search dates	Number and hierarchy of studies included	Intervention types (i.e., community health workers)
Norris, 2006[10]	Diabetes	SR that includes 8 RCTs; each RCT a single-race group. Minority populations were the target of all studies but 2; majority of participants female and middle-aged.	Unrestricted settings: community health workers could have delivered the intervention in the clinic, home or community setting, in either developed or undeveloped countries.	Yes	No	Generic	Systematic review	1966 to March 2004	18 total: 8 RCTs, 6 before-after studies, 3 non-randomized allocation of treatment and comparison groups, 1 study with postintervention measures only	Community health workers serving in a variety of roles
O'Malley, 2003[17]	Preventive	Latino and white patients	Primary care settings (community health clinic or doctor's offices)	Yes. A few included studies are single-race.	Yes. Some included studies are comparative, but do not analyze pre-post by race.	Generic	Systematic review	January 1985-January 2003	n=14 RCT n=5 non-randomized controlled trial n=3 pre-post n=3 quasi-experimental n=3	Clinical reminders; peer health educators; culturally sensitive videos; audit with feedback; vouchers
Osei-Assibey, 2010[24]	Preventive	Adults (18 and older), African Americans, Hispanics, Japanese-Americans and white Americans	All 19 included trials conducted in the US, though not specified if in community or health care settings.	Yes. Most included studies are single-race.	Yes. Some included studies are comparative.	Generic	Systematic review	not specified	N=19 all RCT	Culturally tailored advice/diet counseling; individual programs; family/group programs; peer discussion groups; web-based program;
Peek, 2007[8]	Diabetes	42 studies in which minority patients were >50% racial makeup, or subgroups of larger trials that were specifically described.	Patient education settings included academic primary care clinics and community based health centers. Provider intervention settings included public hospital academic general internal medicine clinics and community based private physician practices. Health care organization interventions occurred in rural and urban locations, academic and community based primary care clinics, and a public hospital diabetes clinic.	Yes. Most included studies are single-race.	Yes. Some included studies are comparative, but the majority do not analyze pre-post by race.	Generic	Systematic review	1985-2006	22 RCTs, 7 RCTs, 13 before/after studies, 1 observational study.	Systematic review of patient-target interventions that sought to improve dietary habits, physical activity, or self-management activities; physician provider-target interventions; health care organization interventions; and multi-target interventions. Included culturally tailored programs. Many health care organization interventions used a registered nurse for case management and/or clinical management via treatment algorithms, often with a CHF for peer support and community outreach. 2 studies evaluated pharmacist-led medication management and patient education. Multi-target interventions involved more than one of the above targets, e.g. multidisciplinary teams.
Perez-Escamilla, 2008[26]	Preventive	Latinos in the US	Community and health care settings	Yes.	No.	Tailored	Systematic review	Not specified	n=22 RCTn Pre-post n=13 Cost-benefit n=1 RCTs: 2 in diabetes peer counseling; 2 breastfeeding; 1 food nutrition education Pre-post: 7 in diabetes peer counseling; 2 in breastfeeding; 5 in food nutrition education	Peer educators; nutrition education; nurse case management
Powe, 2010[19]	Preventive	Individuals aged 50+ and had a study sample of at least 50% African Americans	primary care settings and community based settings	Yes. A few included studies are single-race.	Yes. Most included studies are comparative, but do not analyze pre-post by race.	Generic	Systematic review	2000-2008	n=12 RCT n=8 Nonrandom n=4	Mailed personalized materials; reminder letters/calls; physician reminders; case manager calls; lay health advisors; tailored phone education; physician education

Interventions to Improve Minority Health Care and Reduce Racial and Ethnic Disparities

Evidence-based Synthesis Program

Author, Year, EN ID	Clinical topic	Population	Setting	Single-race (included only minority study participants)	Comparative (included minority and majority participants with pre and post intervention comparison)	Mostly generic or tailored interventions?	Study methodology (e.g., systematic review, meta-analysis)	Study period/search dates	Number and hierarchy of studies included	Intervention types (i.e., community health workers)
Sarkisian, 2003[11]	Diabetes	Studies were in single-race groups only. 2 studies were aimed at older adults and did not specify race.	Various: 1 urban hospital, 2 VAs, 1 rural NOS, 1 in Sweden, 1 in Cuba, others named by city NOS.	Yes	No	Generic	systematic review	Jan 1985 - Dec 2000	8 RCTs 3 Uncontrolled trials using a before/after design 1 RCT but results were presented using before/after analysis	Self-care interventions that aimed to change the behavior of patients, rather than simply educating them. 4 studies were designed according to cultural criteria specific to the targeted group. Techniques for cultural tailoring included focus groups, and using specific recipes for the ethnic group being studied.
Saxena, 2007[9]	Diabetes	US populations in 4 studies. Two studies included both African Americans and Hispanics, and 1 study included only African Americans. 1 study appears to have included only Hispanic African Americans.	Primary Care	No	Yes. Some included studies are comparative, but do not analyze pre-post by race.	Generic	systematic review	Database inception to December 2006	9 studies (4 in UK, 4 in US, 1 in Netherlands). The 4 US studies included 2 RCTs and 2 CCTs.	Primary care interventions, including case management, patient counseling, and reminder cards to prompt providers
Van Voorhees, 2007[34]	Mental health	Ethnic minorities and whites; all ages.	Mostly primary care clinics.	No	Yes. Some included studies are comparative, but do not analyze pre-post by race.	Tailored	systematic review	1/1995 through 1/2006	20 interventions total. 12 chronic disease management (9 multicomponent (8 RCTs, 1 observational/cohort) + 3 single component (1 RCT + 2 observational/cohort); 7 case management + 4 collaborative care) + 8 tailored (3 treatment programs + 4 preventive interventions + 1 psychoeducation).	Case management by trained layperson, nurse, or social worker. Some ethnic matching.
Ward, 2007[35]	Mental health	Ethnic minority and white women (n = 5027 with 2136 ethnic minorities)	PCPs, MH clinics, WIC and other targeted service clinics	No	Yes	Generic	Systematic review	1981 through 2005	10 studies (7 RCTs, 1 observational retrospective design, 1 case series, 1 unclear).	QI, case management, guideline-based interventions, collaborative care, standard psychotherapies, cultural adaptations to psychotherapies.
Webb, 2008[21]	Preventive	African American and whites	Clinical and community	No	Yes	Generic	Meta-analysis	1984-April 2006	n=20 Studies coded as quasi-experimental or RCT, but not reported	Pharmacological (sustained-release bupropion, nicotine patches, nicotine lozenge); individual, phone and group behavioral counseling; targeted print materials; community outreach; video/radio media; multicomponent of above
Webb, 2010[22]	Preventive	healthy US Hispanic adults	Home visits, health care settings, community settings	Yes	No	Generic	Systematic review and mini meta-analysis	1991-2007	n=17 n=12 for SR RCT n=5 for MA	Self help; nicotine replacement therapy; community based interventions; individual counseling; group counseling; telephone counseling
Whitt-Glover, 2009[23]	Preventive	African Americans	Community (churches, YMCA, community centers, public housing) and health care settings (doctor offices, hospitals)	No	Yes	Generic	Systematic review	September 2002-December 2006	n=29 (additional n=14 on children are not considered here) RC=NCT=4 (non-randomized controlled trials-UCT=10 (uncontrolled trial)	Telephone counseling; peer counselors; structured exercise program; group exercise sessions; unstructured/unsupervised exercise

Abbreviations: CHW – community health worker, CVD – cardiovascular disease, DM – diabetes mellitus, ESP – Evidence-based Synthesis Program, GP – general practitioner, HE – health education, HSR&D – Health Services Research and Development Service, MH – mental health, NOS – not otherwise specified, PCP – primary care provider, RCT – randomized controlled trial, VAMC – VA Medical Center, WIC – Special Supplemental Nutrition Program for Women, Infants and Children

APPENDIX E. REVIEWER COMMENTS AND RESPONSES

Reviewer Number	Comment	Response
Question 1: Are the objectives, scope, and methods for this review clearly described?		
1	Yes.	-
2	Yes.	-
3	Yes.	-
4	No. It appears that the objectives for this review evolved during the review due to lack of literature evidence supporting the initial objective. This results in the somewhat confusing review which seems to stray beyond understanding interventions to reduce disparities. Unfortunately, my interpretation of this is that the actual need for a publication of this type, given the limited literature in the area, should be questioned.	The primary stakeholder and nominator for this review topic was HSR&D. The primary purpose for nominating the topic was to take stock of VA race/ethnicity disparities research efforts and to inform future research. We have attempted to deliver a report that serves this purpose.
4	In regards to methods, While a comprehensive literature search was done, it is not clear how the reviewers selected the articles that were retrieved for full text review. That is, approximately 3400 abstracts were reviewed which resulted in 150 articles that underwent further review. What criteria were used to select the articles for further review was not stated.	We have provided a summary of literature search methods and criteria in the methods section, pointing readers to the detailed inclusion/exclusion criteria specified in Appendix B.
5	Yes.	-
6	Yes.	-
7	Yes. Generally, they are. However, clarification is needed regarding the choice of systematic reviews. Also, there needs to be some reference to broader objectives or goals beyond the two key questions – to inform future research and implementation of interventions – see individual comments in the text of the report for more detail.	We have provided a discussion of works in progress by VA disparities researchers as well as mention of informing future research in the report objectives.
8	Yes.	-
Question 2: Is there any indication of bias in our synthesis of the evidence?		
1	No.	-
2	No.	-
3	No.	-
4	Yes. On Page 8 of the review in the background section, a sentence appears as follows, "The extent to which such intervention research has been conducted in VA populations is unclear, though a review of published studies suggests disparities intervention research in the VA may be lagging behind research of interventions conducted outside of the VA setting." It is surprising to me that such a statement would be made without either some citation of the "review" or more direct evidence that supports the statement. This suggests a bias in the reviewers that the VA has conducted little intervention research.	We believe there is some confusion about our usage of the word "review" in this selected sentence. We were not referring to a particular systematic review but were referring more generally to our review of the published literature in the report as a whole. We have amended this sentence.
5	No.	-

Interventions to Improve Minority Health Care and Reduce Racial and Ethnic Disparities

Evidence-based Synthesis Program

Reviewer Number	Comment	Response
5	Appendix C indicates that the systematic reviews were assessed for selection bias (good). However, how they were assessed for selection bias is not described. Also, Appendix C implies that they were not assessed for other types of potential biases (e.g., how they assessed other types of potential bias of the individual studies included within them).	We appreciate that our quality criteria are not elaborated in detail; however, we provide citations that inform our quality guidelines.
5	The document would benefit from descriptions of methodology utilized to assess the risk of bias of any individual studies included in the primary literature review. The PRISMA guidelines for assessing bias might be helpful. Citation: Liberati A, Altman DG, Tetzlaff J, Mulrow C, Gøtzsche PC, et al. (2009) *The PRISMA Statement for Reporting Systematic Reviews and Meta-Analyses of Studies That Evaluate Health Care Interventions: Explanation and Elaboration.* PLoS Med 6(7): e1000100. doi:10.1371/journal.pmed.1000100	We thank the reviewer for providing PRISMA guideline references. The primary objective of the report is to inform VA stakeholders on the state of interventions research in the VA. We have included these primary studies according to inclusion criteria, as well as with regard to our study quality criteria, as indicated in Appendix C. Additionally, these quality criteria appear consistent with PRISMA guidelines.
5	The following statement on page 11 implies that some poor quality reviews may have been included (e.g., if there was only one review available for a given topic, covering a particular time frame, it was always included; even if poor): "If there were several reviews available for a given topic area covering a similar time frame, we excluded poor quality reviews as defined by previously developed criteria." If it is true, it might be more direct to say that all poor quality reviews were excluded.	We have made this change.
6	No.	-
7	No.	-
8	No.	-
Question 3: Are there any published or unpublished studies that we may have overlooked?		
1	No.	-
2	No.	-
3	No.	-
4	No. I am not aware of other literature that was not reviewed in this report.	-
5	No.	-
5	The Robert Wood Johnson Foundation's Finding Answers: Disparities Research for Change program is currently conducting an evaluation of a provider incentive program designed to improve quality of care and outcomes for African American patients with hypertension. The evaluation is designed to assess the impact of the provider incentive intervention on disparities in the 12 participating VA medical centers. More information, including contact info for the PI, can be found here: http://www.solvingdisparities.org/interventions/baylor	Thank you for the information provided.
6	None that I am aware of.	-
7	Yes. I think there needs to be a discussion of current VA funded intervention research, which includes a number of studies that should be informative.	We thank the reviewer for the suggestion. We have included a discussion of ongoing race/ethnic disparities intervention projects in the Discussion section.

50

Reviewer Number	Comment	Response
8	No. Was the following paper included in any of your reviews? It is such a great disparities intervention trial: Peer Mentoring: A Culturally Sensitive Approach to End-of-Life Planning for Long-Term Dialysis Patients. Erica Perry, MSW, June Swartz, MA, Stephanie Brown, PhD, Dylan Smith, PhD, George Kelly, MSW, and Richard Swartz, MD	Thank you for this suggestion. This study did not get captured in our search because it was published prior to our search date, but it is very relevant to the topic. We have added this study to the section on cultural competence interventions.
Question 4: Please write additional suggestions or comments below. If applicable, please indicate the page and line numbers from the draft report.		
1	Page 1: I would refer to prior work as coming from the "VA HSR&D ESP", not the "Portland ESP".	We have made this change.
1	The distinction between Key Questions 1 and 2 is not particularly useful given the paucity of VA-specific studies, and the flow of the text is much improved by combining VA and non-VA intervention studies according to condition or disease. Suggest that your Executive Summary and Text both take that combined approach.	We thank the reviewer for the comment. Several reviewers had concerns about the wording of the two key questions. Consequently, we have reframed our presentation of Key Questions 1 and 2 to avoid confusion.
1	Page 8: Add "VHA Health System Leadership" as a key stakeholder for this evidence synthesis.	We have made this change.
1	I'm not clear I understand the distinction between "targeted" and "deficit" studies – I believe more explanatory text is needed.	Several reviewers were unclear about our categorization scheme. As a result, we have decided to revamp our taxonomic language for clarity and utility in categorizing existing disparities interventions studies. We hope the new scheme will serve this purpose.
1	Page 29 (and elsewhere): Given the likelihood that multicomponent interventions with at least some community-based effort are needed to address health disparities, what are the implications for study design? Are traditional RCTs really feasible? What is the role of community-based participatory research? Qualitative and mixed-methods designs?	We have added a brief discussion of implications for study design in the Discussion section. It will be important for researchers to conduct well-designed and clearly described interventions in Veteran populations to improve the evidence base. It remains to be determined what specific kinds of designs best address these important research questions.
1	Page 29: It is no longer the case that VHA does not consistently collect race/ethnicity data. It is a requirement of policy. However, it is taking the system some time to "catch up". Suggest contacting Denise Hynes or Steve Wright to get current assessment of the completeness and accuracy of race/ethnicity data.	We thank the reviewer for the up-to-date information on VA data collection activities. We are encouraged to hear that it is now a VA policy requirement to collect race/ethnicity for all Veterans. We have amended the recommendations of the report to reflect these developments.
1	I would not favor the recommendation to create a separate Race/Ethnicity Registry. Race/ethnicity data needs to be included in the VA Corporate Data Warehouse, and our data architecture needs to be configured to allow the flexible generation of specific patient cohorts according the shared characteristics that include race/ethnicity. Larry Mole is leading the effort to establish such design principles, so I suggest you contact him for further detail.	We thank the reviewer for the input, and have removed this recommendation from the report.

Interventions to Improve Minority Health Care and Reduce Racial and Ethnic Disparities

Reviewer Number	Comment	Response
2	I found the report's presentation confusing in a number of ways (detailed below), and the take home message hard to identify and digest. I do recognize that the authors were struggling with a fundamental problem – not much literature on the topic of interest and thus they needed to make an effort to find other literature to speak to the issues of the synthesis.	We thank the reviewer for the comment and acknowledgement of the difficulty of the report task. We have made vast changes in an effort to make the take-home message more clear and digestible.
2	I was not sure why this was referred to as a 'preliminary' review in the Exec Summary background – it seems pretty complete.	We removed reference to the review as "preliminary".
2	Throughout the report, I found it confusing that although the first section was entitled "…Interventions within VA health care settings", studies of veterans and in VA were included in the second section, which was entitled "….Interventions outside VA health care settings".	Several reviewers had concerns about the wording of the two key questions. Consequently, we have reframed our presentation of Key Questions 1 and 2 to avoid confusion.
2	It was not clear to me why in the summary of key question #1 on page 2, results were described which were not statistically significant. The terms used to refer to the strength of the results were also a bit confusing – e.g. "XX intervention 'may' reduce disparities" or "the intervention's impact on disparities is 'uncertain'" – these words were hard to interpret.	We have revised our discussion of the results in Key Questions 1 and 2 to be clearer about the strength of evidence.
2	Under "Cardiovascular Disease Interventions" on page 3, reference is made to smoking cessation interventions in the prior section, but that information did not seem to be there.	Reference to smoking cessation findings from the previous section is omitted in the Executive Summary of Cardiovascular Disease Interventions.
2	Given that there is a lot of reference to the quality of the evidence, e.g. 'good', etc. – seems important to define these terms early in the report, rather than solely in the appendix.	We now introduce our quality criteria from Appendix C in the Methods section.
2	Acronyms need to be defined at first use – e.g. HBPC on page 4 and many others throughout (TKR, etc).	We have made this change.
2	The statement on page 6 that 'Minority recruitment efforts to diversify VA personnel will not be effective without commensurate minority patient data recording" comes out of nowhere – no supporting information prior to that summary statement is provided.	We agree that it is unclear how this recommendation derives directly from the results presented in the report. We have removed this recommendation.
2	Page 9 – second bullet under #1 – should probably clarify that interventions could be oriented towards either process and/or outcome.	We have made this change (#1, bullet 2)
	Under 'setting', should indicate that non-VA settings were included.	For #1, only primary studies involving VA settings were considered; non-VA settings were only considered for systematic reviews discussed in #2.
2	Under #2, in sentence beginning 'In addition' – could add, after 'the following' "approaches to intervention delivery".	We have made the suggested change (#2, sentence starting with "In addition").
2	Page 11, under Key question #1, focused on studies of 'interventions involving multiethnic Veteran populations' – but since these were not necessarily disparities reduction interventions, should probably clarify that. Then, still on page 11, under DM interventions, Summary section, it is mentioned that 5 systematic interventions of interventions in _single race_ populations were reviewed. This is confusing – how can these be relevant to disparities reduction?	We have provided a discussion of our inclusion of single-race and multi-race (comparative) studies as potentially offering indirect and direct evidence of disparities reduction, respectively. This discussion is presented with the taxonomy of intervention studies in the state of intervention research subsection.

Reviewer Number	Comment	Response
2	Page 13 – middle paragraph – a study is described which only kept 13 patients over time – is this making too much of a very, very small study?	We thank the reviewer for bringing this to our attention and have addressed these points.
	Through the report, the tense varies within paragraphs, which makes the text harder to follow. Suggest choosing one tense, past or present, and sticking with it throughout.	
2	Page 17 – Cardiovascular Disease Interventions – it states "no intervention studies were specifically designed to reduce disparities" – so I wondered, "why were they included?"	We agree with the reviewer that these studies do not provide direct evidence of interventions to reduce disparities; however we see value in including studies conducted in single-race populations to assess the state of disparities interventions research and to examine specific interventions that appear promising.
2	I thought the proposed new categorization of approaches to delivering interventions was interesting, and can be helpful to the field in the future.	We thank the reviewer for the encouraging remarks.
3	The organization of both the Executive Summary, as well as the full body of the report was somewhat confusing. In particular, I continually wondered why the results of primary studies involving multiethnic Veteran populations, subsumed by Key Question 1, were summarized and presented under the results for Key Question 2.	We thank the reviewer for the comment. Several reviewers had concerns about the wording of the two key questions. Consequently, we have reframed our presentation of Key Questions 1 and 2 to avoid confusion.
3	Part of the confusion on the presentation of findings for Key Question 1 and 2 seems to be an inconsistency in how Key Question 2 is defined throughout the report. In many sections, the question states that interventions "outside VA healthcare settings" will be assessed, whereas in others, the question states that interventions "not limited to VA healthcare settings" will be assessed.	We have referenced Key Question 2 throughout the document as interventions "not limited" to VA settings.
3	The entire report would benefit from a consistent definition of Key Question 2, and it would benefit from findings from Key Questions 1 and 2 being presented under appropriately labeled sections.	We have made this change.
3	On page 5, paragraph 1, the topic sentence beginning, "Examination of non-VA reviews…."	We have revised this sentence.
3	Throughout the report, I had a difficult time discerning the differences between targeted and deficit third generation research studies. Improvements to increase clarity would be helpful.	We have significantly revised our taxonomic language presented in the report. Specifically, we categorize studies by population included – single-race or comparative studies as potentially offering indirect and direct evidence of disparities reduction, respectively. We also present categorization of intervention types as generic or tailored. This discussion is presented with the taxonomy of intervention studies in the state of intervention research subsection, which we hope is more digestible than the "generic," "tailored" and "deficit" distinctions.
3	On page 6, bottom, 4th bullet, beginning "Integrate the use…." is awkwardly stated and requires better wording for clarification.	We have made this change.

Reviewer Number	Comment	Response
3	I wonder whether the concept of "improving health and healthcare quality" rather than "improving health and healthcare" should be added to the Key Study Questions.	Thank you for this suggestion. We have made this change.
3	Page 10, paragraph 1, the search strategy for Key Question 2 again states, "studies not limited to Patients."	We have kept this reference to "not limited to" consistent throughout the report.
3	The Study Results and Methods do not adequately describe how quality was assessed and factored into the presentation of Results. I realize quality scoring is described in an Appendix, but it is not well integrated into the report.	We have better integrated a discussion of quality ratings in the Methods section and throughout the report.
3	The report still needs to have better integration of citations throughout.	Thank you for this suggestion. We have endeavored to improve the integration of citations in the report.
3	Page 17, bullet 1, line 2, there is a typo, "or" should be "of".	We have made this change.
3	Page 18, first full paragraph, I question whether the study should be kept if no data and purely an opinion piece.	Noted.
3	Page 22, summary paragraph, second sentence, I am not sure what is meant by "are characterized by poor evidence."	We have clarified this sentence.
3	Page 23, third full paragraph, not sure why you used a quote from this article, but none of the others. This does not appear to be objective or evidence-based.	We have edited this paragraph.
3	Page 25, paragraph 1, sentence three, please clarify what is meant by "interpersonal connections between patients and the healthcare system."	We have clarified this sentence.
3	In the Discussion Section, the authors make the point that very few difference in differences studies (AA vs. White, etc.) are performed. A more detailed discussion of the sample size, feasibility, and cost implications of carrying-out a multi-center RCT of this nature would be very informative.	We have provided a discussion of the methodological and practical challenges (sample size, feasibility, cost) involved in providing more robust difference-in-difference study designs, and the advantages of partnering with existing large demonstration projects in order to benefit from large outlays in research efforts.
3	Page 26, paragraph 3, Again, I am having a hard time understanding the difference between target and deficit third generation studies.	We have revised the categorization language for improved clarity.
3	Page 28, paragraph 1, Topic sentence, This concept of CBOCs Networks is not well explained or justified. In particular, how often do CBOCs actually exist where low-income, minority Veterans reside?	We have removed mention of CBOCs in the results section (in Summary of Results Across Interventions) and have instead limited discussion of community based outpatient clinics to the Discussion section, where we elaborate on the ability of CBOCs to increase care access for Veterans in less-populated areas.
3	Page 28, paragraph 3, Last sentence; Please clarify what is meant by "boast a robust primary care personnel base."	We have amended this sentence.

Reviewer Number	Comment	Response
3	Page 28, last paragraph, In addition to comprehensively collecting accurate race data, it will be important to have information on ethnicity, sex, literacy, and SES given the complex interrelationships of these social variables.	We agree with the reviewer's assessment. We have included a brief discussion of the importance of considering patient demographics (e.g., SES, gender and literacy) when designing interventions in the Conceptual Framework section of the Discussion.
3	Page 29, paragraph 1, Topic sentence is not clear and requires revision.	We have made this change.
3	Page 29, paragraph 3 discusses distal health outcomes, but I believe references BP, lipid levels, and hemoglobin A-1C which are actually intermediate outcomes.	We have clarified this sentence.
3	Page 29, bullet 2, not sure how minority recruitment efforts to diversify personnel relates to the actual review. This concept and its background needs to be better explained.	We agree that it is unclear how this recommendation derives directly from the results presented in the report. We have removed this recommendation.
4	I found the organization of the review quite confusing. I read the executive summary and put myself in the place of the end user of such a summary. The summary of findings are organized by the 2 key questions which concern studies of interventions for disparity reduction in VA healthcare settings and results of interventions outside the VA health care setting. Despite this clear organization, much of what is mentioned in the non-VA health care settings actually concerns VA studies. While there is some justification for this that is listed much later and buried in the review, this organization was quite distracting.	We thank the reviewer for the comment. Several reviewers had concerns about the wording of the two key questions. Consequently, we have reframed our presentation of Key Questions 1 and 2 to avoid confusion.
4	Again, when I read the title of this report "Interventions to Reduce Racial and Ethnic Disparities" and then find that the major content of the report concerns articles that frankly are not designed to reduce disparity but only to improve outcomes in minority populations, the actual report is quite disappointing. This may reflect the state of the literature in that there are few studies regarding interventions that are published but if that's the case, again, the actual need for such an extensive report, I think, is questionable.	We thank the reviewer for their very frank comments. We have worked to improve the organization and title of the report to reflect the contents more accurately. However, we do believe there is benefit to assessing the current state of intervention research in the VA and highlight opportunities for improving the evidence base.
4	The reviewers might consider reorganizing this report and changing the title to "Interventions to Improve the Health of Minority Populations" as most of the articles that were reviewed and the statement summarizing patterns that seem to improve outcomes concern this topic.	We have revised the title of the report in response to the suggestion.

Reviewer Number	Comment	Response
5	The report might want to reference work by Tom Sequist in which he presents findings that a) providers are likely to acknowledge the existence of disparities in general, but less likely to acknowledge the existence of disparities in their own health care system/clinic and least likely to acknowledge the existence of disparities in their own patient panel. Thus, the importance of collecting RE(L) data is important not only to identify disparities, but also begin to help providers become more aware of, and open to, the existence of disparities within their own organization and practice. Sequist's work also shows that simply providing providers with data/reports on disparities with their own patients (along with cultural competency training) is, while essential, likely not sufficient to reduce or eliminate disparities. Disparity interventions will likely need to be more intensive in order to have a measurable impact. Citations: 1. *Cultural Competency Training and Performance Reports to Improve Diabetes Care for Black Patients: A Cluster Randomized, Controlled Trial* Ann Intern Med. 2010.152:40-46 2. *Physician Performance and Racial Disparities in Diabetes Mellitus Care* Arch Intern Med. 2008. 168(11):1145-1151 3. *Primary-care Clinician Perceptions of Racial Disparities in Diabetes Care* J Gen Intern Med. 2008. 23(5): 678-684	Thank you for suggesting this body of work by Tom Sequist. We have added the findings from the intervention study (suggested paper #1) to the section on cultural competence interventions and have included some of your suggested phrasing.
5	The recommendations on page 7-8 are strong. However, it is not clear how recruiting a more diverse staff his hindered by the lack of patient-level RE data. Is the recommendation that patient-level RE data is a prerequisite to recruiting a staff that is representative of the patient population?	We thank the reviewer for the encouraging remarks. We agree that it is unclear how this recommendation derives directly from the results presented in the report. We have removed this recommendation.
5	I'm not sure if it is relevant due to my lack of exposure to language disparities in VA populations (or lack thereof), but I wanted to offer the possibility that language may be more of an important factor in VA health disparities than the review assumes. Even if all Veterans speak English, is it possible that many still have a preferred language that is not English? In such cases, these patients might experience a higher quality of care and outcomes if their health care is provided in their preferred language. Also, if families and communities are to be incorporated into specific interventions, or the care system in general, they may require services in their preferred language.	We considered this issue. However, language barriers have not been identified as a concern in published studies in Veteran populations. It may be a topic of interest for future research, particularly given that the family and communities supporting Veterans may be non-English speaking.
5	Also, in this section and perhaps elsewhere, there is an implied assumption that relevant disparities are always between white patients (better care and outcomes) compared to racial/ethnic minority groups (worse care and outcomes). However, relevant disparities may exist in which a minority group has better care and outcomes compared to whites, one minority group has better care and outcomes compared to another minority group, etc. Adler (2006: Appendix D in Examining the Health Disparities Research Plan of the National Institutes of Health: Unfinished Business. Gerald E. Thomson, Faith Mitchell, Monique Williams, Editors, Committee on the Review and Assessment of the NIH's Strategic Research Plan and Budget to Reduce and Ultimately Eliminate Health Disparities; PDF is available from the National Academies Press at: http://www.nap.edu/catalog/11602.html) provides a informative overview of different methods to conceptualize and measure disparities. Different approaches may be relevant for a variety of VA settings.	We thank the reviewer for this nuanced discussion point. Although reverse disparities and disparities between minority ethnic groups are indeed important considerations, the commission of this report is focused on taking stock of intervention studies that have potential for reducing and eliminating disparities for minority Veterans, as identified in the 2007 ESP report. We have not sought to exclude studies comparing multiple minority ethnic groups, and have also described the results of interventions with these study populations in this report.

Reviewer Number	Comment	Response
5	The recommendation to incorporate and evaluate the use of community health worker (CHW) and/or other peer-based interventions can be strengthened by advising the use of focus groups, consisting of the target patient population, to explore what they believe are the relevant characteristics of CHW identity that will be the most helpful/important (e.g., from the same neighborhood/community, same R/E, Veteran status, gender, health status/disease diagnosis). The relevant characteristics may vary widely by patient population and/or VA health center. This may significantly influence the potential impact of a CHW program. In other words, it is not necessarily advisable to standardize what defines CHW status because this may change by the patient population and/or health disparity targeted. Finally, directly involving the target population (and resisting the use of proxies) in the design of any intervention will increase the chances of reducing the targeted disparity.	We thank the reviewer for pointing this out. We have re-worded our recommendation so as not to imply that standardization of interventions is necessary. What we do recommend is for components of interventions to be clearly and fully described to allow for comparison across studies.
5	I found the definitions of "generic", "targeted" and "deficit" at the bottom of page 10, and elsewhere, confusing. My confusion comes partly because the term "targeted" is often used in the wider disparities and QI literature to describe intervention design (not study design). In the context of intervention design, it is often used in conjunction with the term "tailored" (targeted - an intervention that is not designed for a particular population/group, but simply directed at them; tailored - an intervention that is specifically designed to meet specific needs, in a culturally competent manner, of a particular population/group). The individual terms/definitions offered do not seem to be complete and/or encompass more than one concept. How are the terms fully differentiated from one another (e.g., the target populations of the intervention, who receives the intervention –or not, and what process and outcomes are measured –or not)? Perhaps it would be easier to characterize the existing disparities research by study design, what process and outcome variables are measured and the adequacy of the control/comparison group (none, internal, external).	We have significantly revised our taxonomic language presented in the report. Specifically, we categorize studies by population included – single-race or comparative studies as potentially offering indirect and direct evidence of disparities reduction, respectively. We also present categorization of intervention types as generic or tailored. This discussion is presented with the taxonomy of intervention studies in the state of intervention research subsection, which we hope is more digestible than the "generic," "tailored" and "deficit" distinctions.
5	Figure 2 may be more accurate if the arrows for "community health workers" and "care coordination" extend through all spheres, including community, neighborhood and individual/home environments. The definitions of the underlying factors and their contributions to the model are not clear.	We have made the suggested change, and have provided more discussion of the underlying factors in the conceptual framework section.
5	The review contains many important/critical recommendations. I have not taken the time to write about the ones I think are strong and clearly defined. However, I want to acknowledge that they are there and appreciated. Thanks!	We appreciate the reviewer's encouragement.
6	Although their numbers are small in comparison to African American/Hispanic Veterans, efforts should be taken to include Asian/Pacific Islander and American Indian Veterans as these groups experience significant disparities in health outcomes also.	We have included this recommendation in our discussion of Future Research Gaps and Implications for VA Health Care Settings (p. 31 last bulleted item).
7	I've used the comment review option to make extensive comments throughout the report. I'm also attaching a current list of HSR&D funded studies (some have been completed). The abstracts are available through our website and ART.	We have addressed the comments in the tracked-changes copy of the report, and have provided a summary table of ongoing HSR&D funded intervention studies.
8	See attached comments in text.	We have adopted the edits and addressed comments made in the text.

Reviewer Number	Comment	Response
Question 5: *Are there any clinical performance measures, programs, quality improvement measures, patient care services, or conferences that will be directly affected by this report? If so, please provide detail.*		
1	This work will help inform the efforts of the Health Equity Workgroup that has been established by Dr Jesse.	Thank you for the suggestion.
2	I don't think so.	-
5	NIH Conference on the Science of Dissemination and Implementation (http://conferences.thehillgroup.com/obssr/di2012/index.html) and IHI National Forum on Quality Improvement in Health Care (http://www.ihi.org/offerings/Conferences/Forum2011/Pages/default.aspx)	Thank you for suggesting these conferences.
6	Newly established VHA Health Care Equality Work Group – *"chartered to leverage talent across VA to determine what VA's response should be to ensure equity for all Veterans."*	Thank you for the suggestion.
7	HSR&D research funding.	Thank you for the suggestion.
Question 6: *Please provide any recommendations on how this report can be revised to more directly address or assist implementation needs.*		
1	Important to highlight how little is known about what works. Our investments need to be in multiple pilots of innovations rather than huge initiatives.	We thank the reviewer for the suggestion. Our discussion now includes recommendations for enhancing the evidence base by funding future pilot intervention studies.
5	Currently, one of the major hindrances to disseminating promising practices/interventions to reduce disparities is the lack of specific information about intervention implementation and maintenance costs (and cost-benefit analyses). Cost information is critical for obtaining buy-in from organization leadership and payers of healthcare. Therefore, recommendations for future research should include gathering, at minimum, basic start-up and maintenance costs for the intervention being evaluated. Whenever possible, cost-benefit analyses should also be encouraged. Also, the lack of specific information about the intervention design and implementation specifics is a significant obstacle to dissemination and ongoing evaluation of best practices and promising strategies. As the review noted, interventions utilizing community health workers or other peer-based models vary widely in terms of identifying staff/volunteers, training methodologies, supervision methodologies, scope of work with patients (e.g., education, counseling, home interventions) and the degree of integration into the medical team. This lack of necessary details (training protocols, forms, software programming) is inherent in the vast majority of intervention evaluation literature. Whenever possible, the documentation and dissemination of implementation details (including unanticipated challenges and solutions) should be encouraged.	We profusely thank the reviewer for the eloquent discussion of one of our key findings of the report. We have elaborated on these points, per the reviewer's suggestion, in the Future Research and Implications in the Discussion section of the report. Thank you for your insightful comments.
6	See comment in #4.	-

Reviewer Number	Comment	Response
7	The planned follow-up survey should be helpful. But I also think that further discussion of what the health care system is able to do regarding the social determinants (if anything is possible) would be helpful.	We thank the reviewer for making this important point. We have included a discussion of the importance of considering social factors in the delivery of health care (Conceptual Model section of the Discussion). More work needs to be done on how best to incorporate this information to help shape interventions and tailor clinical encounters to improve care and outcomes for minority Veterans.
8	I do have some major comments. You mention in the last review you included studies that were underway without to date results. You only found 5 published studies. I think it would be very important to know how many VA disparities studies have not been publicly reported on and why. You might also include some information about currently underway studies. As an FYI I am hoping my (I think) targeted intervention study that was not funded by the VA but conducted in the VA will soon be accepted for publication. It will probably come out too late to be included in this report.	We have reviewed the abstracts of recently funded and ongoing projects in the HSR&D Equity Portfolio and have added our findings to the Discussion. We agree that it would be useful to understand why VA disparities studies have not been publicly reported and have proposed a qualitative survey that hopes to gather insights on this issue.
8	I never quite understood the taxonomy of 3rd generation studies. You define it three times and I was never sure I got what a deficit study was and how it was different from a targeted study.	We have significantly revised our taxonomic language presented in the report. Specifically, we categorize studies by population included – single-race or comparative studies as potentially offering indirect and direct evidence of disparities reduction, respectively. We also present categorization of intervention types as generic or tailored. This discussion is presented in the state of intervention research subsection, which we hope is more digestible than the "generic," "tailored" and "deficit" distinctions.

Reviewer Number	Comment	Response

8	You need to include a section addressing the methodological challenges of performing intervention studies designed to look at differences in differences. There is a reason there are so few intervention studies of this nature both in and outside of the VA. Differences in differences studies usually require huge numbers to detect significant and clinically meaningful differences in outcomes. They are usually performed with secondary administrative data and include large populations. They have been mostly used to look at the association between policy changes and disparities in quasi-experimental designs. Below are some issues relating to choosing intervention designs.
	a. For example a problem might be much more prevalent in minorities (e.g., poor colon cancer screening) but the intervention helps all people with the problem (e.g., care coordination). You do a study offering colon cancer care coordination to all people who have not been appropriately screened and see no differences between blacks and whites in uptake of screening. That does not mean the intervention would not reduce disparities. To really do a difference in difference study you need to study the entire population (including those who have been screened and those who have not). But this is not feasible. What should you do?
	    i. Well first you do a targeted study showing the program works in the at risk population.
	    ii. Then you do an implementation generic study showing it works in a broad array of patients who are unscreened and that a program of this nature can be implemented.
	    iii. You then convince the VA they should pay for this.
	    iv. Then only after it becomes policy and it is broadly adopted can you do a quasi-experimental study looking at change over time in colon cancer screening by race to determine if the intervention really reduces disparities in colon cancer screening.
	
	Clearly I am being a bit over the top but unless you think your intervention is going to be much more effective in minority groups over the majority population it is very hard to show that an intervention reduces disparities. There are very few interventions that are as effective and race specific as the paper on advanced directives cited earlier. Most interventions work on all people with the problem but as you mention in the report, because of social determinants, more people in minority groups are affected by the problem. I think you made an excellent point about tying interventions to large existing programs like PACT but need to address specifically the methodological difficulties with doing these studies.
		We thank the reviewer for bringing up this important point. We have included a discussion of power implications/methodological challenges for performing the interventions recommended.
		
		We appreciate your careful examination of the methodological design challenges inherent in conducting "optimal" disparities reduction intervention studies. As the reviewer points out, large demonstration projects need to serve multiple purposes, and providing large populations of minority Veterans to conduct intervention demonstration projects seems a good opportunity to do so.

Question 7: Please provide us with contact details of any additional individuals/stakeholders who should be made aware of this report.		
1	Suggest contacting Victoria Davey to get input from the Office of Public Health in VHA. Also, you may wish to speak to Larry Mole at Palo Alto to talk about the Registry/Cohort capabilities of the Corporate Data Warehouse.	Thank you for the suggestion.
2	Robert Jesse, MD, PDUSH, who is convening an Equity Healthcare Working group currently (and Susan Schiffner, who works with him and is coordinating that effort)	Thank you for the suggestion.
3	This report clearly should be made available to the Center for Minority Veterans and to Dr. Jesse's VA Health Equality Work Group.	Thank you for the suggestion.
5	Comments: Thank you for this opportunity.	Thank you for the suggestion.
6	Dr Tracy Gaudet, VHA, Director, Patient Centered Care and Cultural Transformation and Dr Garth Graham, HHS's Director, Office of Minority Health and ExOfficio member of VA's Advisory Committee on Minority Veterans.	Thank you for the suggestion.